Manter and Gatz's
Essentials of Clinical Neuroanatomy and Neurophysiology

edition **6**

Manter & Gatz's
Essentials of Clinical Neuroanatomy and Neurophysiology

edition **6**

SID GILMAN, M.D.

Professor and Chairman
Department of Neurology
The University of Michigan Medical School
Ann Arbor, Michigan

SARAH S. WINANS, Ph.D.

Associate Professor
Department of Anatomy and Cell Biology
The University of Michigan Medical School
Ann Arbor, Michigan

F. A. DAVIS COMPANY • Philadelphia

Library of Congress Cataloging in Publication Data

Manter, John Tinkham, 1910–1968
    Manter & Gatz's essentials of clinical neuroanatomy and neurophysiology.

    Rev. ed. of: Manter and Gatz's essentials of neuroanatomy and neurophysiology, 5th ed./Ronald G. Clark. 1975.
    Includes index.
    1. Neuroanatomy. 2. Neurophysiology. I. Gatz, Arthur John, 1907–1971. II. Gilman, Sid. III. Winans, Sarah. IV. Title. V. Title: Manter and Gatz's essentials of clinical neuroanatomy and neurophysiology. VI. Title: Essentials of clinical neuroanatomy and neurophysiology. [DNLM: 1. Nervous system—Anatomy and histology. 2. Neurophysiology. WL 100 M292e]
QM451.M25   1982   612'.8   81-17437
ISBN 0-8036-4155-9   AACR2

PREFACE TO THE SIXTH EDITION

More than 7 years have elapsed since publication of the 5th edition of this book and in this time a number of advances have occurred in our knowledge of the anatomy and physiology of the nervous system. The present edition has been revised extensively to bring the book up to date. In addition, all of the illustrations have been redrawn to provide greater accuracy and clarity. In revising the text, we have held firmly to Dr. Manter's original objective of providing a short but comprehensive survey of the human nervous system. In the present edition, we have placed greater emphasis upon the physiologic and clinical aspects of the nervous system than in the past. The book has been written chiefly for the beginning student of neuroanatomy and neurophysiology. We hope that it will be useful also to students approaching clinical neurologic problems and for individuals from other branches of medicine interested in refreshing their basic knowledge of the nervous system.

We are indebted to Margaret Brudon for her excellent illustrations and to Christine Young for her support, assistance, and counsel.

Sid Gilman, M.D.
Sarah S. Winans, Ph.D.

PREFACE TO THE FIRST EDITION

This book has been written with the object of providing a short, but comprehensive survey of the human nervous system. It is hoped that it will furnish a unified concept of structure and function which will be of practical value in leading to the understanding of the working mechanisms of the brain and spinal cord. Neither of these two aspects—structure and function—stands apart from the other. Together they furnish the key to the significance of the abnormal changes in function that go hand in hand with structural lesions of the nervous system. The viewpoints of three closely dependent sciences—neuroanatomy, neurophysiology and clinical neurology—are combined and used freely, not with the intent of covering these fields exhaustively, but in the belief that a more discerning approach to the study of the nervous system can be attained by bringing together all three facets of the subject.

To suit the needs of the medical student, or the physician who wishes to review the nervous system efficiently, basic information is presented in concise form. Consequently, it has not been feasible to cite published reports of research from which present concepts of the nervous system have evolved. The planning and arrangement of the chapters are such that whole topics can be covered rapidly. Presenting the subject material to classes in this form allows more time for discussion and review, or, if the teacher desires, for lectures dealing with advanced aspects, than would otherwise be permitted.

For the encouragement and valuable suggestions they have given me, I am indebted to my former colleague, Dr. William H. Waller, Jr., and to Dr. Lester L. Bowles. I am deeply grateful to Mr. A. H. Germagian for executing most of the drawings and diagrams, and to Mr. Richard Meyers for his special assistance with the illustrations.

John T. Manter

CONTENTS

1

INTRODUCTION

NERVE CELLS AND NERVE FIBERS

The *neuron* (nerve cell) is the functional and anatomic unit of the nervous system. Each neuron consists of a *cell body* (perikaryon) containing a nucleus and possessing one to several dozen processes of varying length (Fig. 1A, B). *Dendrites* are branching processes that receive *stimuli* and conduct *impulses* generated by those stimuli *toward* the nerve cell body. Most stimuli affecting nerve cells are chemical messengers or *transmitters* that are secreted from one neuron onto an adjacent neuron. The *axon (axis cylinder)* of a nerve cell is a single fiber extending to other parts of the nervous system or to a muscle or gland. The term *axon,* in a physiologic sense, applies to a fiber that conducts impulses *away* from a nerve cell body. Any long fiber, however, may be referred to as an axon regardless of the direction of conduction.

Many peripheral nerve fibers are encased in a *myelin sheath* and a neurolemma (sheath of Schwann) outside the myelin. The myelin is actually a wrapping of many layers of cell membranes from the same Schwann cell that forms the neurolemma. Each Schwann cell contributes myelin to one segment (or internode) of the axon. Between two adjacent Schwann cell internodes is a small gap called the *node of Ranvier* (Fig. 1E). Some fibers have no myelin sheath but retain a single wrapping of cytoplasm from Schwann cells. These fibers are referred to as unmyelinated fibers.

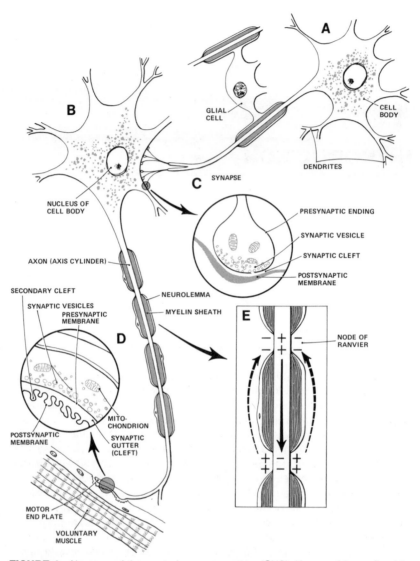

FIGURE 1. Neurons of the central nervous system (CNS). Neuron *A* is confined to the CNS and terminates on neuron *B* at a typical chemical synapse *(C)*. Neuron *B* is a ventral horn cell; its axon extends into a peripheral nerve and innervates a striated (voluntary) muscle at the myoneural junction (motor end plate, *D*). In *E* the action potential is moving in the direction of the solid arrow inside the axon; the dashed arrows indicate the direction of flow of the action current.

The myelinated fibers that are located in the white matter of the brain and spinal cord possess a myelin sheath but have no neurolemma because their myelin sheaths are formed by cytoplasmic extensions of *glial cells,* rather than by Schwann cells. Each glial cell contributes myelin to several nearby axons (see Fig. 1A).

Like all animal cells, nerve cells are enclosed by membranes consisting of lipoprotein bilayers. The intracellular portions of nerve cells contain high concentrations of potassium (K^+) and low concentrations of sodium (Na^+) and chloride (Cl^-) relative to the extracellular fluid, where concentrations of K^+ are low and those of Na^+ and Cl^- are high. These differences in ionic concentrations across nerve cell membranes are maintained by the expenditure of metabolic energy. The result of the differences in the concentrations of these ions (K^+, Na^+, and Cl^-), as well as organic ions, is a difference in electrical potential across the membrane of the nerve cell, with the *inside of the cell strongly negative compared to the fluids outside the cell.* The difference in potential across the membrane is known as the *resting potential.*

Nerve cells are capable of conducting changes in potential along the membranes of both their cell body and the nerve fibers. During impulse transmission there is an alteration of the resting potential and a flow of electrical current across the membrane. The passage of the impulse results from a potential change that commonly is termed the *action potential.* A flow of current occurs during the action potential and is termed the *action current.* The action potential is characterized by a very rapid depolarization (decrease in negativity of the inside relative to the outside) and a somewhat slower repolarization to the resting potential. During the action potential there is a transient reversal of polarity of the electrical potential such that, at the peak of the action potential, the inside of the cell becomes positive with respect to the outside (see Fig. 1E). The action potential results from an initial inward current due to an in-rush of sodium from the exterior to the interior of the cell and an immediately subsequent outward current from the passage of potassium ions from the interior of the cell to the exterior. The passage of ions across the membrane is referred to as an ionic conductance. The conductance of sodium and potassium is thought to occur through separate channels in the cell membrane.

The action potential has characteristics determined only by the properties of the cell, independent of the characteristics of the exciting stimulus. The action potential can be propagated a very long distance along the nerve fiber without any variation of wave form and at an essentially constant velocity. Information within the nervous system is conveyed by the frequency of action potentials rather than the amplitude.

The ability of a nerve cell to produce an action potential is termed *excitability.* The event that elicits an action potential in excitable cells is called a *stimulus.* The minimal stimulus intensity needed to evoke an action potential is termed a *threshold stimulus.* A stimulus below threshold intensity is called *subthreshold* or *subliminal,* and one above threshold intensity is termed *superthreshold* or *supraliminal.* The expression "all or none" is used to describe the ability of a nerve fiber to initiate an action potential with consistent characteristics once a superthreshold stimulus has been applied to its surface. Under some circumstances, subthreshold stimuli may combine to cause an action potential to develop. This process is called *summation*. Summation may result from temporal events, as when two subthreshold stimuli are applied in close succession, or from spatial events, as when two subthreshold stimuli occur simultaneously but at different loci on the neuron.

Nerve cells show *refractoriness,* which is the inability to respond to a second stimulus delivered soon after the first stimulus. During the initial portion of the action potential, triggered by the first stimulus, the cell cannot respond to any other stimulus, no matter how intense. This period is called the *absolute refractory period.* Following the absolute refractory period an action potential can be produced, first by a very intense stimulus, and then gradually by stimuli of lesser intensity. The period after the absolute refractory period is called the *relative refractory period.* In unmyelinated fibers, nerve impulses are propagated through the continuous progression of the action potential along the length of the fiber. In myelinated fibers, the process is the same quantitatively, but there is a major difference. During the propagation of the impulse, the transmembrane ionic current does not flow across the myelin sheath, but flows only across the periodic interruptions of the myelin sheath, which are termed the nodes of Ranvier (see Fig. 1E). As a consequence of myelinization, many fibers that conduct impulses at high velocities can be contained in a relatively small-volume nerve trunk.

Transmission of impulses from neuron to neuron occurs at a synapse (Fig. 1C), which is a place where terminals of the axon of one neuron make contact with the cell body or dendrites of another neuron. Action potentials in the presynaptic neuron cause the release of *neurotransmitters* or neuromodulators from *synaptic vesicles.* The transmitter substance traverses the *synaptic cleft* and either prevents or produces electrical potential changes in the *postsynaptic* neuronal membrane. Ramifications of dendrites and terminal branches of axons form a delicate network throughout the gray matter, known as *neuropil.* Nerve cells normally conduct impulses in only one direction—away from the region that receives stimulation. *Afferent* processes (dendrites) conduct the impulse toward the cell body; *efferent* fibers (axons) conduct away from the cell body.

Nerve cell bodies usually are located in groups. Outside of the brain and spinal cord such groups are called *ganglia.* Within the brain and spinal cord neurons form groups of various sizes and shapes, known as *nuclei.* In this instance the term nucleus has a meaning different from that of the nucleus of an individual cell. The laminated sheets of nerve cells on the surface of the cerebrum and cerebellum are referred to as the cerebral cortex and cerebellar cortex. Regions of the brain and spinal cord that contain aggregations of nerve cell bodies comprise the *gray matter* and, in the fresh state, they are grayish in color. The remaining areas consist primarily of myelinated nerve fibers and make up the *white matter.*

Nerve fibers of the brain and spinal cord that have a common origin and a common destination constitute a *tract.* Although a tract occupies a regular position, it does not always form a compact bundle because of some dispersion with intermingling fibers of neighboring tracts. A number of bundles of fibers in the brain are so distinct anatomically that they have been given the names *fasciculus, brachium, peduncle, column,* and *lemniscus.* These may contain only a single tract, or they may consist of several running together in the same bundle. *Nerve, nerve root, nerve trunk, nerve cord,* and *ramus* are appropriate anatomic terms for bundles of nerve fibers outside the brain and spinal cord.

THE PERIPHERAL NERVOUS SYSTEM

The 12 pairs of cranial and 31 pairs of spinal nerves, with their associated ganglia, make up the human *peripheral nervous system* (PNS). Motor (or efferent) fibers of peripheral nerves are of two types: *somatic motor fibers* that terminate in *skeletal muscle,* and autonomic fibers that innervate *cardiac muscle, smooth muscle,* and *glands.* The termination of the somatic motor fiber on a skeletal muscle fiber occurs at the *motor end plate,* which resembles a synapse (Fig. 1D). The sensory (or afferent) fibers of nerves transmit signals from receptors of various types. Each afferent fiber conducts impulses toward the spinal cord and brain from the particular receptor with which it is connected.

THE CENTRAL NERVOUS SYSTEM

The *central nervous system* (CNS) consists of the brain and the spinal cord. The brain of the young adult human male averages 1380 g in weight (generally 100 g less in females). The adult brain is divided into three gross parts: the cerebrum, the cerebellum, and the brain stem.

The Cerebrum

The left and right cerebral hemispheres are incompletely separated by a deep, *medial longitudinal fissure.* The surface of each hemisphere is wrinkled by the presence of eminences, known as *gyri,* and furrows, which are called *sulci* or *fissures.* The *cerebral cortex* consists of a layer of gray matter that varies from 1.3 to 4.5 mm in thickness and covers the expansive surface of the cerebral hemisphere. This cortex is estimated to contain 14 billion nerve cells.

There are two major grooves on the lateral surface of the brain (Fig. 2). The *lateral fissure (of Sylvius)* begins as a deep cleft on the basal surface of the brain and extends laterally, posteriorly, and upward. The *central sulcus (of Rolando)* runs from the dorsal border of the hemisphere near its midpoint obliquely downward and forward until it nearly meets the lateral fissure. For descriptive purposes the lateral surface of the hemisphere is divided into four lobes. The *frontal lobe* (approximately the anterior one-third of the hemisphere) is the portion which is rostral (anterior) to the central sulcus and above the lateral fissure. The *occipital lobe* is that part lying behind, or caudal to, an arbitrary line drawn from the parieto-occipital fissure to the preoccipital notch. This lobe occupies a small area of the lateral surface but has more extensive territory on the medial aspect of the hemisphere (Fig. 3). The *parietal lobe* extends from the central sulcus to the parieto-occipital fissure and, on the lateral surface, is separated from the *temporal lobe* below by an imaginary line projected from the horizontal portion of the lateral fissure to the middle of the line demarcating the occipital lobe. The gyri within each lobe are subdivided by sulci whose patterns may show considerable individual variation.

Figure 3 depicts the structures that are located on the medial (midsagittal) surface of the brain. This surface is exposed by cutting the brain in half on a plane through the medial longitudinal fissure. This cut severs the corpus callosum, the brain stem, and the cerebellum, and it exposes to view the ventricular system within the brain (Fig. 4). On the medial surface of the cerebral cortex the gyri and sulci of the frontal, parietal, occipital, and temporal lobes are continuous with those seen on the lateral surface. The central sulcus extends a short distance over the dorsal crest of the hemisphere onto the medial side, marking the boundary between the frontal and parietal lobes. The parieto-occipital fissure, as its name implies, separates the parietal and occipital lobes. Only the temporal pole region of the temporal lobe can be seen on this medial section through a whole brain. A part of a fifth lobe can now be seen on the cerebral cortex. This is

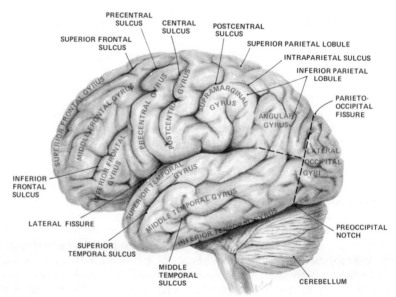

FIGURE 2. Lateral surface of the brain.

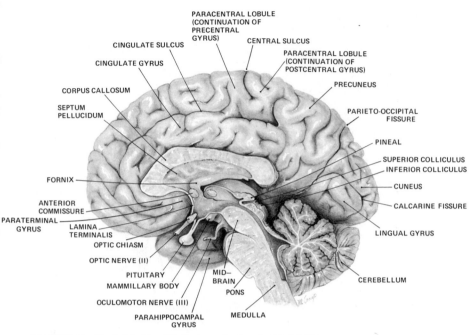

FIGURE 3. Medial (midsagittal) view of a hemisected brain.

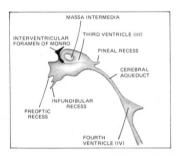

FIGURE 4. Components of the ventricular system as seen on the midsagittal section of the brain (compare Fig. 3).

the *limbic lobe,* a ring (or limbus) of cortical tissue consisting primarily of the paraterminal gyrus, the cingulate gyrus, and the parahippocampal gyrus, which is partially hidden by the brain stem.

A more complete view of the parahippocampal gyrus can be seen on the ventral surface of the brain (Fig. 5). This view also shows the cranial nerves exiting from the brain stem.

A sixth lobe, the *insular lobe,* cannot be seen in any of these figures. It is the cortical tissue that forms the floor of the deep lateral fissure, and can be seen only when the lips (opercula) of this fissure are separated.

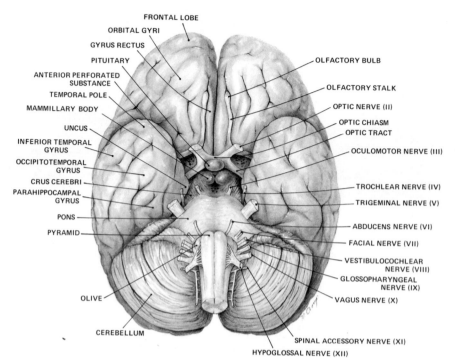

FRONTAL LOBE
ORBITAL GYRI
GYRUS RECTUS
PITUITARY
ANTERIOR PERFORATED SUBSTANCE
TEMPORAL POLE
MAMMILLARY BODY
UNCUS
INFERIOR TEMPORAL GYRUS
OCCIPITOTEMPORAL GYRUS
CRUS CEREBRI
PARAHIPPOCAMPAL GYRUS
PONS
PYRAMID
OLIVE
CEREBELLUM

OLFACTORY BULB
OLFACTORY STALK
OPTIC NERVE (II)
OPTIC CHIASM
OPTIC TRACT
OCULOMOTOR NERVE (III)
TROCHLEAR NERVE (IV)
TRIGEMINAL NERVE (V)
ABDUCENS NERVE (VI)
FACIAL NERVE (VII)
VESTIBULOCOCHLEAR NERVE (VIII)
GLOSSOPHARYNGEAL NERVE (IX)
VAGUS NERVE (X)
SPINAL ACCESSORY NERVE (XI)
HYPOGLOSSAL NERVE (XII)

FIGURE 5. Ventral surface of the brain.

The Cerebellum

The cerebellum is attached to the dorsal surface of the brain stem at the level of the pons. Like that of the cerebral hemispheres, its surface is a layer of gray matter, the cerebellar cortex, which is thrown into ridges and grooves. In the cerebellum the eminences of gray matter are called *folia*. On the midsagittally cut brain (see Fig. 3) a core of white matter, the *arbor vitae,* can be seen under the cortex of the folia.

The Brain Stem

The brain stem consists of the following areas of the brain: *medulla, pons, midbrain,* and *diencephalon.* This region is described in Chapter 9.

THE VENTRICLES, MENINGES, AND CEREBROSPINAL FLUID

Cavities within the brain, called the ventricles, are filled with *cerebrospinal fluid* (CSF). CSF is formed by specialized tissue in the ventricles, called the *choroid plexus.* The ventricular system opens to the space outside the brain at three sites in the brain stem. Through these three openings CSF flows from the ventricles into the *subarachnoid space,* which surrounds the brain and spinal cord. This space exists between the pia mater and the arachnoid, two layers of three connective tissue membranes that enclose the central nervous system. The *pia mater* is intimately attached to the surface of the brain and spinal cord. Fine strands of connective tissue, the trabeculae, stretch across the subarachnoid space between the pia and the *arachnoid.* Outside the arachnoid, the tough *dura mater* lines the bony cranial cavity around the brain and the vertebral canal around the spinal cord. Together, the pia mater, arachnoid, and dura mater constitute the *meninges.* Additional detail on the meninges and CSF can be found in Chapter 25.

THE SPINAL CORD

The human spinal cord is a slender cylinder less than an inch in diameter. It is surrounded by the closely applied *pia mater,* and anchored through the arachnoid to the dura mater by paired lateral septae of pia—the *denticulate ligaments.* From its rostral junction with the medulla to its caudal end, the spinal cord is divided arbitrarily into five regions: cervical, thoracic, lumbar, sacral, and coccygeal. The spinal cord is enlarged in the lower cervical region and in the lower lumbar and sacral regions where nerve fibers supplying the upper and lower extremities are connected. Spinal nerves are attached to the spinal cord in pairs: 8 cervical, 12 thoracic, 5 lumbar, 5 sacral, and 1 coccygeal (Fig. 6). The spinal cord does not extend to the lower end of the vertebral canal but ends at the level of the lower border of the first lumbar vertebra in a tapered cone, the *conus medullaris.* The pia mater continues caudally as a connective tissue filament, the *filum terminale,* which passes through the subarachnoid space to the end of the dural sac (level of vertebra L-5, see Fig. 6), where it receives a covering of dura and continues to its attachment to the coccyx bone. Because the cord is some 25 cm shorter than the vertebral column, the segments of the spinal cord are not aligned opposite corresponding vertebrae. Thus the lumbar and sacral spinal nerves have very long roots extending from their respective segments in the cord to the lumbar and sacral intervertebral foramina where dorsal and ventral roots join to form the spinal nerves. These roots descend in a bundle from the conus and, because of its resemblance to the tail of a horse, this formation is known as the *cauda equina.*

In describing the spinal cord the terms *posterior* and *dorsal* are used interchangeably. Similarly, the terms *anterior* and *ventral* are interchangeable. Sections of the spinal cord cut perpendicular to the length of the cord (transverse sections) reveal a butterfly-shaped area of gray matter with surrounding white matter, which is made up mainly of longitudinal nerve fibers (Fig. 7). Midline grooves are present on the dorsal and ventral surfaces: the *dorsal median sulcus* and the *ventral median fissure.* The lateral surface shows a *dorsolateral* and a *ventrolateral sulcus,* which correspond to the

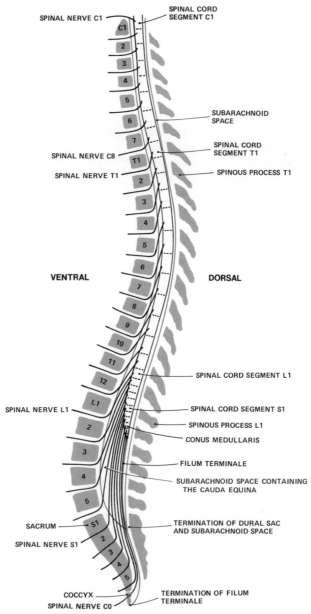

FIGURE 6. Diagram of the relationship of the spinal cord segments and spinal nerve roots to the dural sac and vertebrae of the spinal column. The bodies of the individual vertebrae on the ventral side of the spinal cord are numbered. The spinous processes of the vertebrae are dorsal to the cord. The dural sac and filum terminale are shown in color.

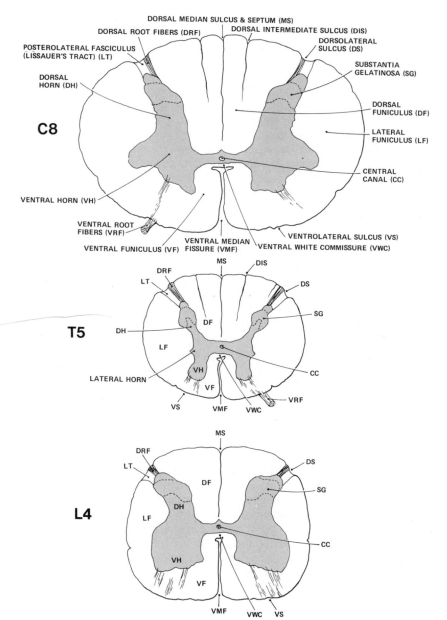

FIGURE 7. Cross sections of the spinal cord at approximately the eighth cervical (C-8), fifth thoracic (T-5), and fourth lumbar (L-4) segmental levels.

dorsal root zone and the ventral root zone respectively. These markings divide the white matter of the spinal cord into *dorsal, lateral,* and *ventral funiculi.* The dorsal root zone is interposed between the dorsal and lateral funiculi, and the ventral root zone is between the lateral and ventral funiculi. The gray matter of the cord contains dorsal and ventral enlargements known as the *dorsal horns* and the *ventral horns.* Small *lateral horns* also are present in the thoracic and upper lumbar segments of the spinal cord (see Fig. 7). The anterior horns are larger in the cervical and lumbosacral enlargements than in the thoracic segments. This is because the muscle mass of the extremities is greater than that of the trunk, and these horns are made up largely of cell bodies of neurons that innervate skeletal muscles. Accordingly, the anterior horn of the lumbosacral enlargement is more massive than that of the cervical enlargement because of the greater muscle mass in the lower extremities. In addition there is more white matter, relative to the amount of gray matter, at cervical levels than in the lumbosacral region (see Fig. 7). This is because the white matter in the cervical region is made up of fibers connecting the entire cord with the brain, whereas the white matter of the lumbosacral cord contains only fibers serving the caudal part of the cord.

In a transverse section of the cord the gray matter can be subdivided into groups of perikarya, called nuclei. When the spinal cord is cut along its length, these nuclei are seen to be cell columns, or laminae. Rexed divided the cord into 10 laminae (Fig. 8). Each lamina extends the length of the cord. Lamina I is in the most dorsal part of the dorsal horn; lamina IX is in the most ventral part of the ventral horn; and lamina X surrounds the central canal. Laminae I through VI are confined to the dorsal horn. Cells here receive and transmit information concerning sensory input from the spinal nerve afferents. Fiber pathways from other cord levels and the brain also influence cells in these laminae. Within laminae I to VI are found several classically defined nuclei or cell columns of the cord. For example, laminae II and III correspond to the *substantia gelatinosa,* which receives information from pain and temperature afferents.

Lamina VII is located in the intermediate gray area and extends into the anterior horn. It contains both the *nucleus dorsalis* and the *intermediolateral gray column.* The connections and functions of these cell groups will be described later. Lamina VIII is located in the ventral horn and contains many neurons that send *commissural* axons to the opposite side of the cord. Lamina IX is restricted to the ventral horn. It contains the *alpha* and *gamma* motoneurons that send axons into the ventral roots of the spinal nerves and innervate the skeletal muscles.

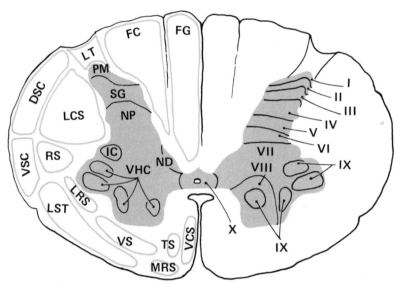

FIGURE 8. Cross section of the spinal cord at approximately the C-8/T-1 segmental level. Tracts and nuclei of the cord are illustrated on the left; Rexed's laminar organization of the gray matter is illustrated on the right. DSC = dorsal spinocerebellar tract; FC = fasciculus cuneatus; FG = fasciculus gracilis; IC = intermediolateral cell column; LCS = lateral corticospinal tract; LRS = lateral reticulospinal tract; LST = lateral spinothalamic tract; LT = Lissauer's tract; MRS = medial reticulospinal tract; ND = nucleus dorsalis; NP = nucleus proprius; PM = posteromarginal nucleus; RS = rubrospinal tract; SG = substantia gelatinosa; TS = tectospinal tract; VCS = ventral corticospinal tract; VHC = ventral horn cell columns; VS = vestibulospinal tract; VSC = ventral spinocerebellar tract.

2

FUNCTIONAL COMPONENTS OF THE SPINAL NERVES

The function of the nerves of the body may be categorized conveniently by the following method: the fibers that innervate the body wall are termed *somatic;* those that innervate the viscera are termed *visceral; sensory* fibers are designated *afferent;* and *motor* fibers are designated *efferent.*

SUMMARY OF FUNCTIONAL COMPONENTS

General Afferent Fibers

General afferent fibers are the sensory fibers that have their cells of origin in the *dorsal root ganglia.* These cells differ significantly in shape from the neurons pictured in Figure 1. Dorsal root ganglia cells are round and have only one process leaving the cell body. That process soon splits into a peripheral process, which enters the nerve, and a central process, which passes through the dorsal root to the spinal cord.

  General somatic afferent (GSA) fibers (Fig. 9) carry exteroceptive information from receptors in the skin mediating pain, temperature, touch, and proprioceptive information from sensory endings in the muscles, tendons, and joints.

  General visceral afferent (GVA) fibers carry sensory impulses from receptors in the visceral structures within the body.

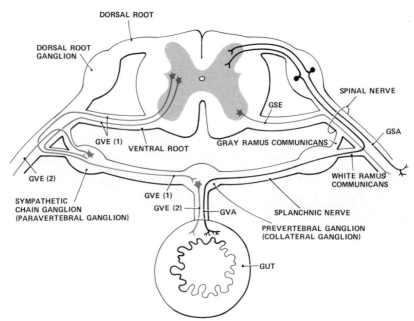

FIGURE 9. Function components of a spinal nerve. General somatic afferent (GSA), general visceral afferent (GVA), and general somatic efferent (GSE) fibers and their cells of origin are illustrated on the right and are arbitrarily separated, for clarity, from the general visceral efferent fibers and cells (GVE-1 and GVE-2) on the left. The autonomic (GVE) structures diagrammed here belong to the sympathetic division.

General Efferent Fibers

General somatic efferent (GSE) fibers consist of the motor fibers, originating from alpha and gamma motoneuron cell bodies of lamina IX, that innervate the striated musculature (derived from the myotomes of somites).

General visceral efferent (GVE) fibers consist of the autonomic fibers that innervate smooth and cardiac muscle and that regulate glandular secretion. *Preganglionic sympathetic* cell bodies are located in the intermediolateral cell column extending from C-8 or T-1 to L-2 (lamina VII). *Preganglionic parasympathetic* cell bodies are located in a similar region in the sacral cord (S-2 to S-4). The axons of these cells are labeled GVE(1) in Figure 9. In the sympathetic ganglia (or parasympathetic ganglia in the pelvis), GVE(1) fibers synapse on the cell bodies of postganglionic autonomic fibers, which are labeled GVE(2) in Figure 9.

CLASSIFICATION OF NERVE FIBERS

Nerve fibers can be categorized according to fiber diameter, thickness of the myelin sheath, and speed of conduction of the nerve impulse. In general, *the greater the diameter of the fiber, the thicker the myelin sheath, and the faster the conduction velocity.* Currently, two classifications of nerve fibers are in use. One is an electrophysiologic classification based upon the conduction velocities of motor and sensory nerve fibers as revealed by peaks in the action potential when an entire compound nerve is stimulated electrically. In this classification, nerve fibers consist of three groups: A, B, and C. The A and B fibers are myelinated, and the C fibers are unmyelinated. A fibers are subdivided further on the basis of mean conduction velocity and, hence, fiber size into several subgroups: alpha, beta, gamma, and delta. C fibers are subdivided into two classes: sC fibers (postganglionic efferent sympathetic C fibers) and drC fibers (afferent dorsal root C fibers). The A fibers contain two important motor components: alpha fibers, which innnervate extrafusal muscle, and gamma fibers, which innervate intrafusal muscle (muscle spindles).

A second classification, pertaining only to sensory fibers, divides the fibers into four groups, chiefly on the basis of fiber size, but also according to fiber origin. Three important elements in this classification are group Ia afferents (spindle primary afferents), which arise in muscle spindles; group Ib afferents, which originate in Golgi tendon organs; and group II afferents (spindle secondary afferents), which come from muscle spindles.

Table 1 summarizes the two classifications.

TABLE 1. Classification of Nerve Fibers

SENSORY AND MOTOR FIBERS	SENSORY FIBERS	LARGEST FIBER DIAMETER	FASTEST CONDUCTION VELOCITY (METERS/SEC)	GENERAL COMMENTS
A-α	Ia	22	120	Motor: the large alpha motoneurons of lamina IX, innervating extrafusal muscle fibers
				Sensory: the primary afferents of muscle spindles
A-α	Ib	22	120	Sensory: Golgi tendon organs, touch and pressure receptors
A-β	II	13	70	Motor: the motoneurons innervating both extrafusal and intrafusal (muscle spindle) muscle fibers
				Sensory: the secondary afferents of muscle spindles, touch and pressure receptors, and Pacinian corpuscles (vibratory sensors)
A-γ	III	8	40	Motor: the small gamma motoneurons of lamina IX, innervating intrafusal fibers (muscle spindles)
A-δ	III	5	15	Sensory: small, lightly myelinated fibers; touch, pressure, pain, and temperature
B		3	14	Motor: small, lightly myelinated preganglionic autonomic fibers
C	IV	1	2	Motor: all postganglionic autonomic fibers (all are unmyelinated)
				Sensory: unmyelinated pain and

3

SPINAL REFLEXES AND MUSCLE TONE

SPINAL REFLEXES

A reflex action consists of a specific, stereotyped response to an adequate stimulus. The stimulus for a spinal reflex involves input to the central nervous system from peripheral receptors, including muscle, skin, and joints. The response usually involves contraction of the striated skeletal muscle fibers (extrafusal fibers). A reflex response may be mediated by as few as two neurons, one afferent and one efferent, and in this case it is termed a monosynaptic reflex response. Muscle stretch (deep tendon) reflexes such as the knee jerk are mediated by monosynaptic reflexes. In most instances, a reflex response involves several neurons, termed interneurons or internuncial cells, in addition to the afferent and efferent neurons. A reflex may involve neurons in (1) just one or a few spinal cord levels, as in the case of segmental reflexes (those restricted to a single spinal cord segment); (2) several to many spinal cord levels, as with intersegmental reflexes; or (3) structures in the brain that influence the spinal cord, as in the case of supraspinal reflexes.

MUSCLE SPINDLES

Muscle spindles are encapsulated structures, 3 to 4 mm in length, located in varying numbers in most skeletal muscles of the body (Fig. 10). They are particularly numerous in the small, delicate muscles of the hand. A spindle consists of 2 to 12 thin muscle fibers of modified striated muscle. Because they are enclosed in the fusiform spindle, they are termed intrafusal muscle fibers to contrast them with the large extrafusal fibers. The muscle spindle is attached to the connective tissue septae that run between extrafusal fibers. Consequently, the entire muscle spindle structure is connected in parallel to the extrafusal fibers, a fact that is important in the function of the muscle spindle. There are two distinct types of intrafusal fibers, as well as a third, intermediate type. The longer and larger fiber contains numerous large nuclei closely packed in a central bag and hence is called a nuclear bag fiber (see Fig. 10). The other type is shorter and thinner and contains a single row of central nuclei. The structure resembles a chain and thus is known as a nuclear chain fiber (see Fig. 10). A third, recently recognized type of muscle spindle intrafusal fiber is intermediary in structure between bag and chain fibers.

Both bag and chain fibers are innervated by gamma motoneurons which terminate in two types of endings—plates and trails (see Fig. 10). Plate endings occur chiefly on nuclear bag fibers and rarely on nuclear chain fibers. Trail endings occur mostly on nuclear chain fibers but are found frequently on bag fibers as well. Muscle spindles are amply supplied with sensory nerve endings of two types: primary endings derived from group Ia nerve fibers and secondary endings derived from group II fibers. Primary afferents arise in the central equatorial region of both bag and

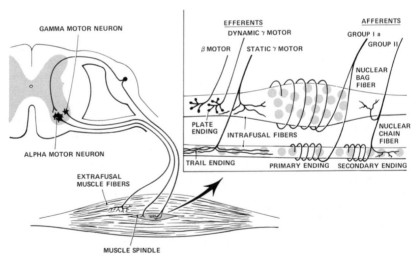

FIGURE 10. A cross section of the spinal cord showing a Ia afferent fiber originating in a muscle spindle, passing through a peripheral nerve, entering a dorsal root, and making synaptic connection with an alpha motoneuron. The axon of the alpha motoneuron emerges through the ventral root, passes through the peripheral nerve, and terminates in the extrafusal muscle fibers. The axon of the gamma motoneuron makes synaptic connection with the intrafusal fibers of the muscle spindle. The inset shows an enlarged view of the muscle spindle with its principal endings.

chain fibers. Secondary endings arise predominantly on nuclear chain fibers and lie to either side of the primary endings.

ALPHA AND GAMMA MOTONEURONS

Muscle contraction in response to a stimulus, in the final analysis, must involve activation of the alpha and gamma motoneurons of lamina IX. Alpha motoneurons are the largest of the anterior horn cells. They can be stimulated monosynaptically by (1) the Ia primary afferents and group II secondary afferents of the muscle spindles; (2) corticospinal tract fibers in primates; (3) lateral vestibulospinal tract fibers; and (4) reticulospinal and raphe spinal tract fibers. Although alpha motoneurons can be stimulated monosynaptically, in a vast majority of cases they are stimulated through interneurons in the spinal cord gray matter in response to reflex activation of segmental, intersegmental, and supraspinal circuits. All descending tracts of the spinal cord ultimately influence the activity of these neurons. Alpha motoneurons innervate not only the large extrafusal skeletal muscle fibers, but also interneurons (Renshaw cells) through collateral fibers emerging from the axons of alpha motoneurons. Renshaw cells are capable of inhibiting alpha motoneurons, producing a negative feedback response. This can have the beneficial effect of turning off the alpha motoneuron immediately after it has fired so that it will be able to fire again.

Gamma motoneurons, which are also termed fusimotor neurons, innervate the intrafusal muscle fibers within the muscle spindles of skeletal muscle. They do not innervate extrafusal muscle fibers and, consequently, do not produce extrafusal muscle contraction. Gamma motoneurons differ from alpha motoneurons in other ways as well: (1) they are smaller; (2) they are not excited monosynaptically by segmental inputs; (3) they are not involved in inhibitory feedback mechanisms by Renshaw cells; and (4) they tend to discharge spontaneously, often at high frequencies. Despite these differences between gamma and alpha motoneurons, both generally respond similarly to incoming stimuli. Most of the descending pathways of the spinal cord influence the activity of both types of neurons. The reticular system, cerebellum, and basal ganglia exert particularly strong control over the gamma motoneurons. Beta motoneurons innervate both extrafusal and intrafusal muscle fibers.

THE STRETCH REFLEX

The stretch reflex is the basic neural mechanism for maintaining tone in muscles. Aside from its role in keeping relaxed muscles slightly active, the stretch reflex is capable of increasing the tension of select muscle groups to provide a background of postural muscle tone on which voluntary movements can be superimposed.

The stretch (myotatic) reflex can be tested by tapping the tendon of a muscle such as the patellar tendon. This stretches the extrafusal fibers of the quadriceps femoris muscle group. Since the intrafusal fibers are arranged in parallel with the extrafusal fibers of the quadriceps, the muscle spindles also will be stretched. The stretching stimulates the sensory endings in the spindles, particularly the primary afferents (group Ia fibers). The Ia afferents stimulate monosynaptically the alpha motoneurons that supply the quadriceps muscle and inhibit polysynaptically the antagonistic muscle group (the hamstring muscles). Consequently, the quadriceps suddenly contracts and the hamstring muscles relax, causing the leg to extend at the knee.

The sensory function of the intrafusal fibers is to inform the nervous system of the length and rate of change in length of the extrafusal fibers. In the absence of any gamma motoneuron activation, the primary afferents respond to both the length of muscle and the rate of change in length of muscle. In contrast, the secondary endings respond chiefly to muscle length. Activation of gamma motoneurons makes the intrafusal muscle fibers contract and therefore makes the sensory portion of the muscle spindles more responsive to stretch. Since muscle spindles are located in parallel with extrafusal fibers, muscle spindles shorten during muscle contraction and this results in cessation of discharge of the afferent nerve fibers. Gamma motoneuron activation can prevent muscle spindles from ceasing to fire during extrafusal muscle contraction. Activation of gamma motoneurons also makes the muscle spindles more responsive to stretch.

Two types of gamma motoneurons have been described. One type affects the afferent responses to phasic stretch more than the responses to static stretch. This group is called the *dynamic gamma motoneurons.* The other type increases the spindle response to static stretch and thus is called the *static gamma motoneurons.* Dynamic gamma motoneurons are thought to terminate in plate endings solely on nuclear bag fibers, whereas static gamma fibers terminate in trail endings on both bag and chain fibers. Gamma motoneurons thus can adjust the length of intrafusal fibers so that the spindle receptors can always operate on a sensitive portion of their response scale. In addition, during a powerful contraction with considerable shortening, it may be advantageous for the spindle receptors to continue firing in order to reinforce the power of the contraction reflexly. This is referred to as the *servo-assisted* method of producing and controlling movement. Much of the information from spindles is utilized at high levels of the nervous system, particularly the cerebellum and cerebral cortex. These regions can influence the descending pathways that facilitate and inhibit alpha and gamma motoneuron activity. Supraspinal, intersegmental, and segmental influences tend to cause the discharge of both alpha and gamma motoneurons innervating a particular muscle. This phenomenon is known as *coactivation.*

Group Ia fibers innervating the primary endings in muscle spindles establish direct monosynaptic connections with alpha motoneurons innervating the same (homonymous) muscles and synergistic (heteronymous) muscles. Group II afferent fibers from muscle spindles excite homonymous alpha motoneurons monosynaptically.

GOLGI TENDON ORGANS

Golgi tendon organs are encapsulated structures located in series with the large, collagenous fibers of tendons at the insertions of muscles and along the fascial covering of muscles. Within the capsule, sensory nerve endings (Ib afferents) terminate in small bundles of collagenous fibers of tendons. When muscle contraction occurs, shortening of the contractile part of the muscle results in lengthening of the noncontractile region where tendon organs are located. The result is vigorous firing of the Golgi tendon organs. Thus these receptors are primarily sensitive to muscle contraction. Their central action is to inhibit polysynaptically the alpha motoneurons innervating the agonist muscle and to facilitate motoneurons of the antagonist muscle. The central actions of the Golgi tendon organs are responsible for the "clasp-knife" phenomenon in spasticity, which is described below.

MUSCLE TONE

The term *muscle tone* indicates the resistance that an examiner perceives when manipulating passively the limbs of a patient. In the relaxed normal subject, when a limb is manipulated at one of the joints, a certain amount of resistance will be encountered in muscle that is not related to any conscious effort on the part of the patient. There are two general abnormalities of muscle tone, termed hypotonia and hypertonia. Hypotonia is a decrease of resistance to passive manipulation of the limbs, and hypertonia is an increase of resistance to passive manipulation of the limbs.

Hypotonia occurs in a limb at once if the ventral roots containing the motor nerve fibers to the limb are cut. Hypotonia also results from transection of the dorsal roots that contain sensory fibers from the muscle. Thus muscle tone is maintained and regulated in muscles by reflex activity of the nervous system and is not a property of isolated muscle. Hypotonia may occur also with disease affecting certain parts of the nervous system, particularly the cerebellum. Hypertonia appears in one of two general forms—spasticity and rigidity. In spasticity there is an increase in the resistance to passive manipulation of the "clasp-knife" type, and this is usually accompanied by an increase of the deep tendon reflexes. The "clasp-knife" phenomenon indicates a marked increase of resistance to passive manipulation (in flexion or extension), occurring during the initial portion of the manipulation. As the manipulation proceeds, the resistance suddenly decreases and disappears. In rigidity there is a plastic or a "cogwheel" type of resistance to passive manipulation, often without changes in the deep tendon reflexes.

REFLEXES OF CUTANEOUS ORIGIN

The sensory receptors in skin and subcutaneous tissues respond to touch, pressure, heat, cold, and tissue damage. These receptors generate signals that have reflex effects on spinal motoneurons mediated by interneurons.

The flexor and crossed extensor reflexes are examples of aversive responses that permit a limb to be withdrawn from a source of injury and that allow a postural compensation to occur. A noxious stimulus to a limb results in flexion of the ipsilateral limb and extension of the contralateral limb. A common example occurs when an individual steps on something very hot or sharp. This results in reflex withdrawal of the stimulated extremity. It is due to the polysynaptic facilitation of alpha motoneurons innervating the ipsilateral flexor muscles with inhibition of motoneurons innervating the extensor muscles of the same leg. Simultaneously, the opposite limb extends in order to support the weight of the body. The limb extension results from facilitation of motoneurons innervating extensor muscles and inhibition of motoneurons innervating flexor muscles.

4

THE DESCENDING PATHWAYS

MOTOR AREAS OF THE CEREBRAL CORTEX

The *primary motor area,* also known as Brodmann's area 4, is located in the precentral gyrus of the frontal lobe (see Figs. 2 and 50). It extends from the lateral fissure upward to the dorsal border of the hemisphere and a short distance beyond on the medial surface of the frontal lobe in the rostral aspect of the paracentral lobule (see Figs. 3 and 51). The left motor strip controls the right side of the body and the right strip, the left side. The larynx and tongue are influenced by neurons in the lowest part of this strip, followed in upward sequence by the face, thumb, hand, forearm, arm, thorax, abdomen, thigh, leg, foot, and the muscles of the perineum. The neurons controlling leg, foot, and perineal muscles are in the paracentral lobule. In humans, areas for the hand, tongue, and larynx are dispropor-tionately large, conforming with the development of elaborate motor control of these muscle groups. A functional map of the motor cortex resembles a distorted image of the body turned upside-down and reversed left for right (see Fig. 52). Immediately rostral to area 4 is the *premotor cortex,* which consists of *areas 6 and 8.* Area 8 influences eye movements. The most medial aspect of area 6 can be observed on a midsagittal section of the brain just rostral to the paracentral lobule (see Fig. 51). This is the location of the *supplementary motor area.* A third motor area is found in the *postcentral cortex* (areas 3, 1, and 2 of Brodmann). Another motor area, referred to as the *secondary motor area,* is present on the most ventral aspect of the precentral and postcentral gyri near the lateral fissure. This overlaps the *secondary somatosensory cortex* (see Fig. 53). The functions of the supplementary and secondary motor areas are unclear.

DESCENDING FIBERS FROM THE CEREBRAL CORTEX AND BRAIN STEM THAT INFLUENCE MOTOR ACTIVITY

Skeletal muscle activity is the result of the net influence upon the alpha and gamma motoneurons of the spinal cord and upon the motor components of the cranial nerve nuclei. Collectively, these are the neurons that provide the final direct link with muscles through myoneural junctions (motor end plates). Such neurons are referred to as lower motoneurons (LMN). Their cell bodies reside within the central nervous system, and their axons make synaptic contact with extrafusal and intrafusal muscle fibers of somatic and branchiomeric origin. *Somatic* muscle fibers derive from true somites in the developing embryo. *Branchiomeric* muscles stem from segments of the head and neck, which develop into gill arches in water-dwelling verte-brates. These branchiomeres are not true somites, but the muscles which develop from them, like somatic muscles, are striated and under voluntary control.

A number of descending motor pathways regulate lower motor neu-ronal activity, which, in turn, controls somatic and branchiomeric muscles. These descending pathways are controlled directly or indirectly by the ce-rebral cortex, cerebellum, or basal ganglia. In the strictest sense, the neu-rons in all such pathways should be referred to as *upper motoneurons* (UMN). Upper motoneurons operate directly, or through interneurons, upon alpha and gamma motoneurons and upon motor components of the cranial nerve nuclei. They are contained completely within the central nervous system. Clinicians usually use the term UMN only when referring to the corticospinal tract or, to a lesser extent, the corticobulbar tract (Fig. 11).

Corticospinal Tract

The corticospinal tract, also termed the pyramidal tract, was once consid-ered to be the pathway that initiated and controlled all "voluntary" muscu-lar activity. It is now known to be concerned primarily with skilled move-ments of the distal muscles of the limbs and in particular with facilitation of the alpha and gamma motoneurons that innervate distal flexor muscula-ture. Approximately one-third of the axons in this tract arise from area 4, the primary motor cortex, and about 3 percent of these fibers originate from unusually large pyramidal cells, called Betz cells, which are located in the fifth layer of the cortex. Another one-third of the fibers arise from area 6, and the remainder of the fibers originate from the parietal lobe (primarily areas 3, 1, and 2 of the postcentral gyrus).

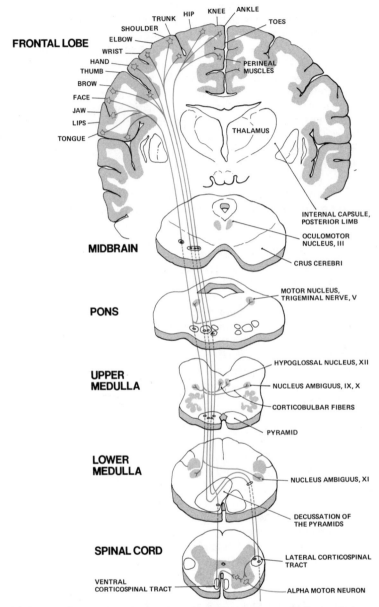

FIGURE 11. The corticospinal and corticobulbar pathways of the central nervous system.

The corticospinal tract passes through the posterior limb of the internal capsule and the middle of the crus cerebri (see Fig. 11). It then breaks up into bundles in the basilar portion of the pons and finally collects into a discrete bundle, forming the pyramid of the medulla. This pathway was originally named the pyramidal tract because of its passage through the medullary pyramid, and not because of its origin from pyramidal cells in the cortex. In the lower levels of the medulla, most of the corticospinal tract crosses (decussates) to the opposite side. This region is referred to as the level of the motor or pyramidal tract decussation. Approximately 90 percent of the fibers cross at this level and descend through the spinal cord as the *lateral corticospinal tract,* which passes to all cord levels in the lateral funiculus and synapses in the lateral aspect of laminae IV through VIII. Many of the cells in these laminae are interneurons which, in turn, synapse on alpha and gamma motoneurons in lamina IX. In primates a small percentage of the fibers (perhaps those arising from Betz cells) synapse directly upon the alpha and gamma motoneurons in lamina IX. These motoneurons innervate the muscles in the distal parts of the extremities (hands and feet).

The 10 percent of corticospinal fibers that do not decussate in the medulla descend in the anterior funiculus of the cervical and upper thoracic cord levels as the *ventral corticospinal tract.* However, at their respective levels of termination, the fibers in this pathway decussate through the anterior white commissure prior to synapsing upon interneurons and motoneurons. The number of fibers in both lateral and ventral corticospinal tracts decreases in successively lower cord segments as more and more fibers reach their terminations.

The corticospinal tract is not purely motor. It also sends fibers to synapse on interneurons in laminae IV, V, and VI of the spinal cord. These interneurons, in turn, can influence local reflex arcs and cells of origin of ascending sensory pathways. Thus the cerebral cortex can control motor output and also modify sensory input reaching the brain.

Corticobulbar Tract

The fibers of the corticobulbar tract arise from neurons in the ventral lateral part of areas 4 and 6, and from area 8. The axons start out in company with the corticospinal tract but take a divergent route at the level of the midbrain (see Fig. 11). A few of the fibers continue along with the corticospinal tract into the pyramids. The fibers of this pathway terminate in the brain stem where they influence (but not by direct, or monosynaptic, connections) the motor nuclei of cranial nerves III (oculomotor); IV (trochlear); V (trigeminal); VI (abducens); VII (facial); IX, X, and XI (glossopharyngeal, vagus, and accessory); and XII (hypoglossal). Fibers from cortical area 8, the frontal eye fields, influence eye movements indirectly by synapsing on cells in the superior colliculus, pretectal nuclei, and accessory optic nuclei of the midbrain. These areas, in turn, project directly, or via another relay in the paramedian pontine reticular formation, to the nuclei of cranial nerves III, IV, and VI. Corticobulbar fibers from the face region of areas 4 and 6 terminate on interneurons adjacent to the motoneurons that innervate the remaining striated skeletal musculature, either of somatic or branchiomeric origin. With the exception of the portion of the facial nucleus that innervates facial musculature below the angle of the eye, the cranial nerve motor nuclei are innervated bilaterally, and the muscles that they control cannot be contracted voluntarily on one side only. The lower facial nucleus receives innervation from the opposite cerebral cortex only (see Fig. 33). Clinical evidence indicates that sometimes the hypoglossal nucleus receives only a crossed component.

Like the corticospinal tract, the corticobulbar tract contains fibers that terminate on sensory "relay" neurons. In the brain stem these relay nuclei include the nuclei gracilis and cuneatus, the sensory trigeminal nuclei, and the nucleus of the solitary fasciculus.

Corticotectal Tract

In the past, some authors have used the term "corticomesencephalic tracts" to identify the pathways that arise from cerebral cortical areas 18 and 19 in the occipital lobe and project to the upper parts of the brain stem to influence extraocular muscle movement. These fibers are referred to here as the corticotectal tract. Many of the fibers synapse in the superior colliculus, the interstitial nucleus of Cajal, or the nucleus of Darkschewitch. These nuclei, in turn, project through the paramedian pontine reticular formation and the medial longitudinal fasciculus (MLF) to synapse upon the oculomotor, trochlear, and abducens nuclei. Other cortical fibers may first synapse in various regions of the reticular formation that influence the extrinsic eye muscle nuclei directly or via connections through the MLF.

Corticorubral and Rubrospinal Tracts

The corticorubral and rubrospinal tracts represent an indirect route from the cerebral cortex to the spinal cord. Fibers originating from the same cortical areas that give rise to the corticospinal tract form the *corticorubral tract*. This tract projects to the ipsilateral red nucleus in the tegmentum of the midbrain. The red nucleus gives rise to the *rubrospinal tract*, a crossed pathway that is found in the spinal cord just anterior to the lateral corticospinal tract in the lateral funiculus (see Fig. 8). Its fibers synapse at all cord levels in the lateral aspect of laminae V, VI, and VII and thus overlap part of the termination of the corticospinal tract. In fact, the rubrospinal tract is functionally similar to the corticospinal tract in that it facilitates flexor and inhibits extensor alpha and gamma motoneurons, particularly those innervating the arms. The red nucleus is also a way station between the cerebellum and the ventral lateral nucleus of the thalamus.

Corticoreticular and Reticulospinal Tracts

The reticular formation (a matrix of nuclei in the core of the brain stem) receives a large input from *corticoreticular fibers*, which accompany the corticospinal tract. Two areas of the reticular formation send major projections into the spinal cord. The pontine reticular formation gives rise to the uncrossed *pontine (medial) reticulospinal tract.* In the brain stem this pathway travels just ventral to the medial longitudinal fasciculus. In the spinal cord it passes through the ventral funiculus (see Fig. 8) to all cord levels. Its fibers synapse in laminae VII and VIII. This tract is mainly facilitatory for extensor motoneurons, particularly those innervating the legs, and provides an important input to gamma motoneurons. The medial aspect of the medullary reticular formation gives rise to the *medullary (lateral) reticulospinal tract,* which is primarily uncrossed but has a small crossed component. This tract passes to all cord levels in the lateral funiculus just anterior to the rubrospinal tract. There is controversy regarding the exact function of this pathway with respect to the alpha and gamma motoneurons. It synapses in laminae VII and IX. The tract conveys *autonomic information* from higher levels to the preganglionic sympathetic and parasympathetic neurons to influence respiration, circulation, sweating, shivering, and dilation of the pupils, as well as the function of the sphincteric muscles of the gastrointestinal and urinary tracts.

Raphe-Spinal and Ceruleus-Spinal Projections

Fibers arising from neurons within the raphe nuclei, particularly the nucleus raphe magnus, project to the spinal cord through the dorsolateral funiculus. These fibers terminate within laminae I, II, and V, ending upon preganglionic sympathetic neurons as well as other neurons. The raphe-spinal projection is serotonergic and appears to be involved in pain mechanisms.

The nucleus locus ceruleus and nucleus subceruleus give rise to a projection descending into the spinal cord through the lateral funiculus and terminating in laminae I, II, V, VII, IX, and X. This projection is noradrenergic.

Vestibulospinal Tracts

The two vestibulospinal tracts are discussed in Chapter 14. Both of these tracts pass into the anterior funiculus and synapse upon cells in laminae VII and VIII. The lateral *vestibulospinal tract* extends the entire length of the cord, and the *medial vestibulospinal tract* extends only to upper thoracic levels. The lateral tract facilitates extensor alpha motoneurons and inhibits flexors. In some mammals, the medial vestibulospinal tract sends inhibitory fibers directly to the upper cervical alpha motoneurons. This is an unusual situation. In most other systems, inhibition of motoneurons is mediated through inhibitory interneurons.

Medial Longitudinal Fasciculus

The medial longitudinal fasciculus (MLF), as its name implies, is not a single tract but a bundle of several tracts, some of which project into the ventral funiculus of the spinal cord. This "descending portion" of the MLF contains the *pontine reticulospinal tract* and the medial *vestibulospinal tract,* which have already been discussed. In addition, it contains the *tectospinal tract,* which arises from the superior colliculus and crosses to the opposite side near the oculomotor nucleus (in the dorsal tegmental decussation) to join the MLF. The *interstitiospinal tract,* which arises from the interstitial nucleus of Cajal (an accessory oculomotor nucleus), is also part of the MLF. It supplies only the upper cervical levels where it synapses in laminae VII and VIII. The MLF is concerned with neck and head reflex movements in response to visual and vestibular stimuli.

THE INFLUENCE OF DESCENDING PATHWAYS UPON THE SPINAL CORD

The motor system pathways arising in the cerebral cortex and brain stem that reach the spinal cord consist functionally of two general groups. At the level of the brain stem, these pathways can be divided into ventromedial and lateral groups. The ventromedial group consists of fibers arising in the vestibular and reticular nuclei that project to the spinal cord through the lateral vestibulospinal and the medullary and pontine reticulospinal tracts. These tracts terminate in the ventral and medial aspects of the anterior horn of the spinal cord, including laminae VII and VIII. The ventromedial pathways are concerned in particular with maintenance of the erect posture, integrated movements of the body and limbs, and progression movements of the limbs. These pathways generally tend to facilitate the activity of motoneurons projecting to extensor muscles and to inhibit the activity of motoneurons projecting to flexor muscles.

The lateral pathway consists of fibers arising in the red nucleus that project to the spinal cord through the rubrospinal tract. This pathway terminates in the dorsal and lateral aspect of the anterior horn of the spinal cord, including laminae V, VI, and VII. The lateral pathway is concerned with fine manipulative movements of the limbs, particularly the hands and feet. This pathway generally facilitates the activity of motoneurons projecting to flexor muscles and inhibits the activity of motoneurons projecting to extensor muscles. The corticospinal projections mediate controls similar to those of the lateral pathway, but also provide the capacity for fine manipulative movements of the fingers.

Clinicians usually divide the descending pathways into pyramidal and extrapyramidal groups. The pyramidal pathway consists of the corticospinal fibers that course through the medullary pyramid, and the extrapyramidal pathways consist of all the other descending pathways.

5

PAIN AND TEMPERATURE

The sensations of pain and temperature are mediated by the anterolateral system, which consists of a diffuse bundle of fibers located at the junction of the anterior and lateral funiculi of the spinal cord. The cells of origin of the anterolateral system are activated by dorsal root afferents including A-δ and C fibers as well as larger myelinated cutaneous afferents. The system contains pathways which include the lateral and ventral spinothalamic tracts. Other components of the pathway, mainly spinoreticular, do not reach the thalamus and thus cannot be termed "spinothalamic." Axons of the anterolateral system arise from cells located in several layers of the dorsal horn. Most of these axons cross through the ventral commissure of the spinal cord and ascend, though a small number may ascend ipsilaterally. This system conveys itching and tactile sensations in addition to pain and temperature. The tactile components will be considered in Chapter 7.

THE DORSAL ROOTS

Essentially all sensations are conveyed into the central nervous system by the dorsal roots, which consist almost entirely of sensory or afferent nerve fibers. A small number of sensory fibers have been discovered in the ventral roots. Many of these fibers respond to painful superficial or deep stimuli, but their function is uncertain. The cell bodies of the dorsal root fibers are located in the spinal, or dorsal root, ganglia. Each ganglion cell possesses a single nerve process which divides in the form of a "T" with a central branch running to the spinal cord and a peripheral branch coming from a receptor organ (Fig. 12). There are no synapses in a spinal ganglion. The area in which the dorsal root fibers enter the spinal cord, in the region of the dorsolateral sulcus, is called the dorsal root zone. There is a tendency for the largest and most heavily myelinated fibers to occupy the most me-

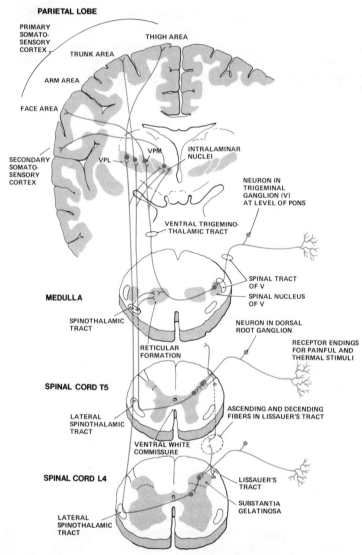

FIGURE 12. The central nervous system pathways mediating the sensations of pain and temperature.

dial position in this zone and the small myelinated and unmyelinated fibers the most lateral.

THE PAIN-TEMPERATURE PATHWAYS

The peripheral receptors for pain are thought to be the naked terminals of fine nerve fibers. Many of them may be specialized chemoreceptors that are excited by tissue chemicals released in response to noxious stimuli. The stimulus that evokes pain is usually intense and may cause destruction of, or damage to, tissue. Neural responses to noxious stimuli are mediated by A-δ and C peripheral nerve fibers that enter the spinal cord through the lateral part of the dorsal root zone and divide at once into short ascending and descending branches that run longitudinally in the posterolateral fasciculus (Lissauer's tract). Within a segment or two, these fibers leave this tract to make synaptic connections with neurons in the dorsal horn, including interneurons in laminae I, II and III (substantia gelatinosa), IV, and V. These interneurons project to neurons in laminae V through VIII and there make synaptic connection upon the cells of origin of the anterolateral system, including the lateral and ventral spinothalamic tracts and the spinoreticular projections.

The axons of spinothalamic tract cells cross anterior to the central canal in the *ventral white commissure* and then course rostrally in the *anterolateral funiculus.* The lateral spinothalamic tract extends through the spinal cord and brain stem, supplying inputs to the *reticular formation,* the *superior colliculus,* and several *thalamic nuclei,* including the *intralaminar nuclei,* the *posterior nuclear complex (PO),* and the *ventral posterolateral nucleus (VPL),* referred to by physiologists as part of the *ventrobasal complex.* Thalamocortical fibers relay pain information from the thalamic nuclei primarily to the *secondary somatic sensory area* of the cerebrum (see Figs. 12 and 53). Some fibers conveying painful and thermal sensations from the VPL nucleus also may project to the *primary somatosensory cortex*—areas 3, 1, and 2 of the postcentral gyrus (see Figs. 12, 50, and 51). Like the adjacent primary motor cortex, the somatosensory cortex is organized by body parts. The fibers from the upper parts of the body project to cortical areas near the lateral fissure, and the fibers conveying information from the lower limb and perineum terminate on the medial surface of the hemisphere, in the paracentral lobule (see Fig. 53).

Portions of the anterolateral system are phylogenetically old. The system consists of the "paleospinothalamic tract," which projects to the medial portions of the thalamus, and the "neospinothalamic tract," which projects to the ventral posterolateral region of the thalamus. These two pathways, in conjunction with the spinoreticular projections, constitute the anterolateral system. The anterolateral system is predominantly a slowly conducting, polysynaptic system. In humans, a small percentage of the fibers go directly to the thalamus, but most synapse in the medial aspect of the reticular formation throughout its length in the brain stem. Ascending reticular fibers, in turn, relay pain information to thalamic nuclei and to the hypothalamus and limbic system. The projection of the anterolateral system to the VPL nucleus is organized somatotopically so that the input from the upper body is located medial to that from the lower body (see Fig. 12).

Pain fibers from the face, the cornea of the eye, the sinuses, and the mucosa of the lips, cheeks, and tongue are carried in the *trigeminal nerve* and its sensory ganglion (the semilunar, trigeminal, or gasserian ganglion). Upon entering the brain stem in the pontine region, these fibers form a descending tract, the *spinal tract of V.* Terminals of the spinal tract of the trigeminal nerve form synapses in an adjacent nucleus, the *spinal nucleus of V.* Axons originating in the spinal nucleus of V cross to the opposite side and ascend as the *ventral (anterior) trigeminothalamic tract* to the *ventral posteromedial nucleus (VPM)* of the thalamus (see Fig. 12). This pathway also projects to the reticular formation and the medial and intralaminar thalamic nuclei that receive projections from the anterolateral system. The cortical projections of the VPM are to the part of the somatosensory cortex closest to the lateral fissure. The areas of the body most sensitive to somatosensory stimuli (e.g., lips and fingers) have disproportionately large areas of neuronal representation in the somatosensory cortex.

PERCEPTION OF PAIN

Although the clinical management of pain is a problem that confronts the physician continually, there are wide gaps in our knowledge concerning the structure and function of the receptors and central pathways mediating this modality. Pain is composed of a distinctive sensation and the individual's reaction to this sensation with accompanying emotional overtones, activity in both somatic and autonomic systems, and volitional efforts of avoidance or escape. Three types of pain sensation are generally recognized. The first is "fast" pain, consisting of a sharp, pricking sensation that is accurately localized and results from activation of A-δ fibers, which are myelinated. The second is a burning pain, which has slower onset, greater persistence, and less clear location. "Slow" pain results from activation of C fibers, which are unmyelinated. The third type of pain is described as aching, sometimes with a burning sensation, and results from stimulation of visceral and deep somatic receptors. These receptors are connected with nerve fibers running largely in sympathetic and somatic pathways consisting of both unmyelinated and A-δ sized myelinated afferent fibers.

There is no convincing evidence that separate central nervous system pathways mediate "fast" pain or "slow" pain. There is good evidence that the neospinothalamic pathway, projecting to the ventral posterolateral nucleus of thalamus and to somatosensory areas I and II in the cerebral cortex, is essential for the spatial and temporal discrimination of painful sensations. The paleospinothalamic pathway and the spinoreticular pathway mediate the autonomic and reflexive responses to painful input, and probably the emotional and affective components of pain.

Painful stimuli apparently can be detected at the level of the thalamus, in the absence of the cerebral cortex. In humans, destruction of the posterior and intralaminar nuclei has been found to relieve intractable pain. However, such lesions may be effective only briefly and pain may return. Although this point is controversial, it appears that destruction of the cerebral cortical somatosensory projection areas in the postcentral region does not eliminate pain. Lesions of the mediodorsal nucleus of the thalamus, or transection of the fibers linking this nucleus to the frontal lobe ("prefrontal leukotomy"), can diminish the anguish of constant pain by changing the psychological response to painful stimuli. Marked changes in personality and intellectual capacities occur with these lesions. The posterior portions of the cerebral hemisphere, including the parietal lobe, are responsible for appreciating the localizing qualities of pain and integrating painful modalities with other types of sensory stimuli.

ENKEPHALINS AND ENDORPHINS

Electrical stimulation of peripheral nerve fibers or of discretely distributed loci in the brain can elicit analgesia. Recent studies have shown that the analgesia from electrical stimulation of the central nervous system probably results from the release of morphine-like substances called enkephalins. The enkephalins are naturally occurring substances that bind to the same receptors in the central nervous system that bind opiate drugs. Enkephalins are thought to be transmitters in specific neural systems of the brain. These transmitters and their opiate-binding receptors are found in the brain structures involved in modulation of pain transmission by the administration of opiate drugs. One of these transmitter systems is concentrated densely in the dorsal horn, particularly in laminae I to III. The effect of enkephalin release and binding upon their receptors is a suppression of the activity of neurons in the immediate vicinity. This is thought to be a mechanism by which pain may be suppressed.

Electrical stimulation of the midline raphe nuclei of the brain stem can induce analgesia in experimental animals. The raphe nuclei are found throughout the brain stem, and their axons descend to the spinal cord through the dorsolateral fasciculus. The axons terminate in the dorsal horn where they attenuate the responses of spinothalamic and other dorsal horn cells to noxious stimuli.

The endorphins are short-chain neuropeptides found chiefly in the pituitary gland but also in the brain. These substances have a high affinity for the opiate receptors of the brain and pituitary gland and have been reported to elicit analgesia when injected into the brain.

TEMPERATURE SENSE

The receptors in the skin for the sensations of cold and warmth consist of naked nerve endings. The peripheral nerve fibers mediating these sensations consist of the thinly myelinated A-δ and some C fibers. Other types of

C fibers mediate only the painful components of the extremes of heat and cold stimulation. The central nervous system pathway for thermal sensation appears to follow the same course as that of the pain pathway. The two systems are so closely associated in the central nervous system that they can scarcely be distinguished anatomically, and injury to one usually affects the other to a similar degree.

EFFECT OF CUTTING THE LATERAL SPINOTHALAMIC TRACT

The lateral spinothalamic tracts are sometimes sectioned in humans to relieve intractable pain—a surgical procedure known as tractotomy. The cut is made in the anterior part of the lateral funiculus. Some damage is done to the ventral spinocerebellar tract, and perhaps to certain extrapyramidal motor fibers, but no permanent symptoms are produced except a loss of pain sensibility on the contralateral side, beginning one or two segments below the cut (see Fig. 16). In some patients pain is relieved only temporarily, suggesting that other routes may be available or that the information is mediated by both crossed and uncrossed tracts. Bilateral tractotomy is usually necessary to abolish pain from visceral organs.

SENSORY EFFECTS OF DORSAL ROOT IRRITATION

Mechanical compression or local inflammation of dorsal nerve roots irritates pain fibers and commonly produces pain which is felt along the distribution of the roots affected. The area of skin supplied by one dorsal root is a dermatome, or skin segment. The approximate boundaries of human dermatomes are shown on the left side of Figures 13 and 14. Pain that is limited in distribution to one or more dermatomes is known as radicular pain. Peripheral fibers of each spinal nerve branch, and these branches join those of adjacent spinal nerves to form *peripheral nerves.* The cutaneous branches of each peripheral nerve therefore carry fibers from more than one spinal nerve, and the skin territory of each of these peripheral nerves covers portions of several dermatomes (see Figs. 13 and 14, right side).

Sensory changes other than pain may be associated with dorsal root irritation. There may be localized areas of paresthesia, such as spontaneous sensations of prickling, tingling, or numbness. Zones of hyperesthesia, in which tactile stimuli appear to be grossly exaggerated, may be present. If the pathologic process is a progressive one that gradually destroys fibers, the dorsal roots will finally lose their ability to conduct sensory impulses. There will then be hypesthesia (diminished sensitivity) and eventually anesthesia (the complete absence of all forms of sensibility).

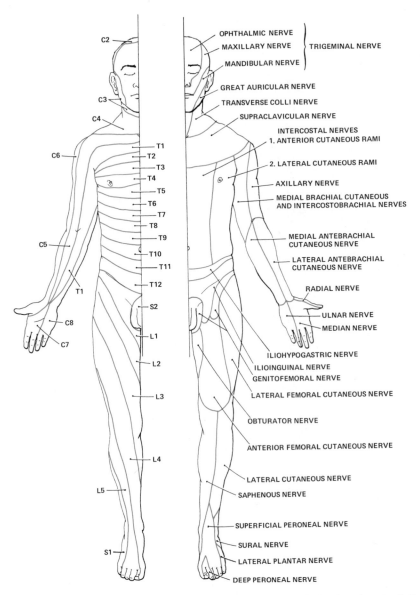

FIGURE 13. The innervation of the front surface of the body by dorsal roots *(left)* and peripheral nerves *(right)*.

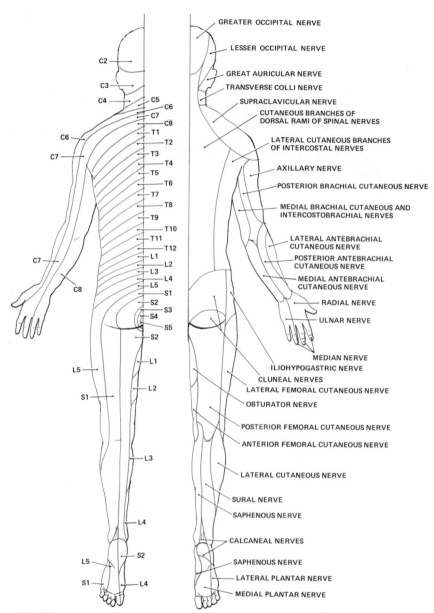

FIGURE 14. The innervation of the rear surface of the body by dorsal roots *(left)* and peripheral nerves *(right)*.

VISCERAL REFERRED PAIN

The parenchyma of internal organs, including the brain itself, is not supplied with pain receptors. However, the walls of arteries, all peritoneal surfaces, pleural membranes, and the dura mater covering the brain may be sources of severe pain, especially when they are subjected to inflammation or mechanical traction. Abnormal contraction or dilation of the walls of hollow viscera also causes pain.

Pain of visceral origin is apt to be vaguely localized. At times it is felt in a surface area of the body far removed from its actual source, a phenomenon known as *referred pain*. For example, the pain of coronary heart disease may be felt in the chest wall, left axilla, or down the inside of the left arm; inflammation of the peritoneum covering the diaphragm may be felt over the shoulder. In each case, the neurons that supply the skin area in which the pain is felt enter the same segment of the spinal cord as do the neurons that actually conduct the pain stimuli from the visceral organ. Spinal cord segments T-1 and T-2 receive sensory fibers from skin areas of the left upper extremity and from the heart as well; segments C-3, C-4, and C-5 supply the skin of the shoulder area and also receive sensory fibers from the diaphragm. One of the many theoretical explanations of referred pain is that the visceral sensory fibers are discharging into the same pool of neurons in the spinal cord as the fibers from the skin, and that an overflow of impulses results in misinterpretation of the true origin of the pain.

Pain may be referred from deep somatic structures. In the case of ligaments and muscles associated with the vertebral column, the referred area is not always in the same segmental distribution as the level of origin of the pain impulses.

6

PROPRIOCEPTION AND STEREOGNOSIS

THE LEMNISCAL SYSTEM

The term "lemniscal system" is used commonly to differentiate a component of the somatic afferent system that is separate from the anterolateral pathway. The lemniscal system begins with receptors that send information to the CNS about muscle stretch, the position and movements of joints, and vibratory, tactile, and pressure stimuli on the skin. The receptors include muscle spindles and Golgi tendon organs as well as Pacinian corpuscles and other encapsulated receptors in muscles, tendons, ligaments, and joints. These are the proprioceptors, and the information they provide is essential for awareness of the position of the limbs and their movements, often referred to as kinesthetic sense. Most of these receptors are innervated by large-diameter myelinated fibers. The cell bodies of these peripheral nerve fibers are in the dorsal root ganglia, and their central processes enter the medial side of the dorsal root zone. The fibers enter the spinal cord and travel within the ipsilateral dorsal column, terminating in the dorsal column nuclei (nuclei gracilis and cuneatus). Many fibers of the lemniscal system travel within the lateral column as well as the dorsal column, and thus the term *dorsolateral pathway* is used for the spinal portion of the lemniscal system. The dorsal column nuclei send projections to the ventrolateral portions of the thalamus, and this nucleus projects to the postcentral gyrus of the cerebral cortex.

The lemniscal system is organized to provide information about the location, spatial form, and temporal sequences of somatic stimuli. The ability to appreciate these stimulus qualities is termed *stereognosis:* recognition of the form of objects with stimulation on the skin. Information concerning these sensations is relayed not only to the level of the cerebral cortex, but also to certain subcortical sites, particularly the cerebellum, where the information is used for motor control and not sensation.

PATHWAYS OF PROPRIOCEPTION AND STEREOGNOSIS AND THE SPINOCEREBELLAR PROJECTIONS

After entering the spinal cord, proprioceptive fibers and fibers from mechanoreceptors continue without synaptic interruption in at least three divergent routes (Fig. 15).

Direct Fibers to Lower Motoneurons in the Ventral Gray Horns

These are the afferent fibers of the two neurons (afferent and efferent) that make up the stretch reflex arc. They arise within muscle spindles and end in synaptic contact with alpha motoneurons within a few spinal segments of the level at which they enter the spinal cord (see Fig. 10).

Fibers to Spinocerebellar Pathways

Some proprioceptive fiber collaterals (primarily from Ia and Ib afferents) as well as many fibers conveying other sensory modalities such as touch, pressure, and pain synapse with neurons in the base of the posterior horn of the cord (see Fig. 15). Neurons within several laminae at lumbar and sacral levels send primarily crossed fibers to the *ventral spinocerebellar tract,* the most peripheral tract in the ventral margin of the lateral funiculus.

The *nucleus dorsalis,* or *Clarke's nucleus* (lamina VII), located in the base of the dorsal horn (T-1 through L-2), receives Ia and Ib afferents from muscle spindles, Golgi tendon organs, and joint receptors and sends ipsilateral fibers rostrally in the *dorsal spinocerebellar tract,* which is located just posterior to the ventral spinocerebellar tract in the lateral funiculus. The dorsal and ventral spinocerebellar pathways are primarily concerned with the lower extremities. The dorsal spinocerebellar tract provides information concerning individual extremity muscles and joints, whereas the ventral spinocerebellar tract relays information from pain, tactile, and pressure receptors over the extremity.

Some fibers from the levels of C-1 to T-5 travel up the dorsal funiculus (fasciculus cuneatus) to synapse with neurons in the *accessory cuneate nucleus.* This nucleus is the upper extremity counterpart of Clarke's nucleus and gives rise to the ipsilateral *cuneocerebellar tract (dorsal arcuate fibers).* All of the above tracts terminate primarily in the midline portion

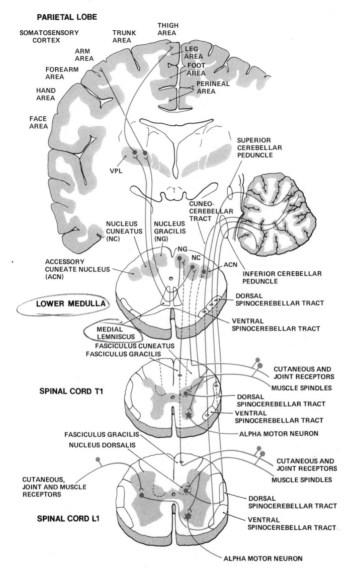

FIGURE 15. The central nervous system pathways mediating proprioception and stereognosis.

(vermis) of the cerebellar cortex. The dorsal spinocerebellar and cuneo-cerebellar tracts enter the cerebellum through the inferior cerebellar peduncle. The ventral spinocerebellar tract takes a separate course and enters the cerebellum through the superior cerebellar peduncle (Fig. 15). These tracts report the ongoing activity of muscle groups to the cerebellum. The latter is thus capable of modifying the action of the muscle groups so that the resulting movements are smoothly and accurately performed. The forelimb equivalent of the ventral spinocerebellar tract is the rostral spinocerebellar tract (not shown in Figure 15).

The spinocerebellar pathways are not considered to be part of the lemniscal system.

Fibers Turning Directly Upward in the Posterior Funiculus

The fibers that form the first link of a pathway carrying proprioceptive information to the cerebrum arise from receptors for position sense, which are found in the connective tissue near joints. Recent evidence suggests that fibers from muscle spindles (Ia fibers) and Golgi tendon organs (Ib fibers) may also project through this system to the thalamus and contribute to position and movement sense. These fibers ascend in the posterior funiculi of the spinal cord to relay nuclei in the lower part of the medulla. Fibers from the leg ascend adjacent to the dorsal median septum and form the *fasciculus gracilis* (see Fig. 15). Fibers from the arm ascend lateral to the leg fibers and constitute the *fasciculus cuneatus.* Both fasciculi ascend to the lower medulla where they terminate in the *nucleus gracilis* and *nucleus cuneatus* respectively. Clinicians often refer to these tracts as the posterior or dorsal column pathways and to the nuclei as the dorsal column nuclei. As mentioned earlier, because of recent evidence that the lateral column of the spinal cord also mediates proprioceptive information, the lemniscal pathway in the spinal cord should be termed the dorsolateral pathway. Fibers from the cells of the dorsal column nuclei promptly cross to the opposite side in the decussation of the medial lemniscus. They then ascend as the *medial lemniscus* to the thalamus and terminate in the *ventral posterolateral (VPL) nucleus.* In contrast to the anterolateral system discussed in the last chapter, few, if any, of the fibers in this system synapse in the reticular formation. Thalamocortical fibers from the VPL continue to the *postcentral gyrus* of the parietal lobe. The band of the cortex that receives these terminals has been designated as the somesthetic area or somatosensory cortex. The topographic representation of the body areas in this region is similar to that of the motor strip which lies parallel with it on the opposite side of the central sulcus. The conscious recognition of body and limb posture requires cortical participation.

In addition to fibers mediating proprioception, other fibers concerned with certain aspects of the senses of touch, pressure, flutter-vibration, and kinesthesis travel in the posterior funiculi, medial lemnisci, and thalamus to the postcentral gyri. This pathway appears to be important in providing information about the place, intensity, and temporal and spatial patterns of neural activity evoked by mechanical stimulation of the skin, particularly moving stimuli. This pathway to the cerebral cortex is necessary for discriminative tactile sensation. Tactile discrimination has several components, including two-point discrimination (the ability to appreciate two separate points at which pressure is applied simultaneously); stereognosis (the ability to recognize the size, shape, and texture of objects by palpation); and complex tactile discrimination (tested, for example, by having a patient identify letters and figures drawn on the skin). The lemniscal system is responsible also for the sense of limb position and movement, including the sense of steady joint angles, the sense of motion produced by active muscular contraction (kinesthesis) or passive movement, the sense of tension exerted by contracting muscles, and the sense of effort. In addition, the lemniscal system is responsible for the sense of flutter-vibration. The sense of flutter is a feeling of repetitive movement, and the sense of vibration is a more diffuse and penetrating feeling of humming when a vibrating tuning fork is held in contact with a bony prominence on the body.

The Lateral Cervical System

The lateral cervical system mediates touch, vibratory, and proprioceptive senses as well as nociceptive sensation. It is described in Chapter 7.

DISTURBANCES OF SENSATION FOLLOWING INTERRUPTION OF THE LEMNISCAL PATHWAYS

Complete loss of proprioceptive sensation from a spinal lesion requires interruption bilaterally of the dorsolateral pathway (both dorsal columns and the medial part of the dorsolateral columns). The results of lesions in this location are deficits in position sense, vibration sense, and tactile discrimination. The symptoms occur prominently on the same side of the body after unilateral injury of a dorsolateral funiculus (Fig. 16). Symptoms are also found, in varying degrees, with lesions of the gracile and cuneate nuclei, the medial lemniscus, the thalamus, and the postcentral gyrus. Lesions of the lemniscal pathway leave preserved the sensations of pain and temperature. Interruption of the dorsal columns without injury to the lateral columns results in deficits of fine and rapid conscious adjustments of position and loss of detection of the direction of a moving stimulus, but touch and movement sense remain intact.

Clinical signs of injury to the lemniscal pathways, frequently tested in a neurologic examination, include the following:

1. Inability to recognize limb position. The patient is unable to say, without looking, whether a joint is put in a position of flexion or extension. The patient also cannot detect the direction of limb displacement during a movement.
2. Astereognosis. There is loss, or impairment, of the ability to recognize common objects, such as keys, coins, blocks, and marbles, by touching and handling them with the eyes closed.
3. Loss of two-point discrimination. There is loss of the normal facility of recognizing two points simultaneously applied to the skin as dis-

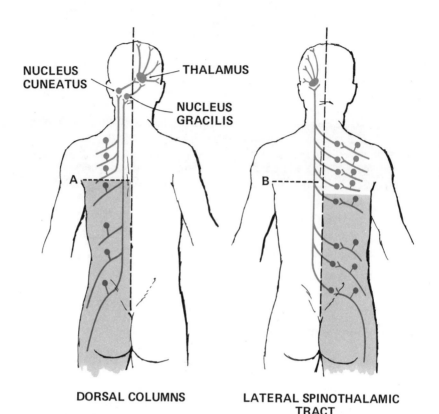

NUCLEUS
CUNEATUS

THALAMUS

NUCLEUS
GRACILIS

A

B

DORSAL COLUMNS

LATERAL SPINOTHALAMIC
TRACT

FIGURE 16. The shaded regions show the body surface areas affected by interrupting the dorsal column on the left (A) and the lateral spinothalamic tract on the right (B). In A the sensory disturbance is on the ipsilateral side of the body because the ascending fibers cross above the level of the lesion, in the medulla. In B the sensory loss is on the contralateral side of the body and one or two segments below the level of the lesion because fibers entering the lateral spinothalamic tract ascend one or two segments and then cross to the opposite side of the body.

tinct from a single point. The two points of a compass may be used for testing, though the tips of the compass should be blunt.

4. Loss of vibratory sense. The sensation evoked by a vibrating tuning fork applied by the base to a bony prominence is normally perceived as mildly tingling. When this ability is lost, the patient cannot differentiate a vibrating fork from a silent one.

5. Positive Romberg sign. In this test the patient is asked to stand with his feet placed close together. The amount of body sway is noted while the eyes are open, then compared with the degree of sway present with the eyes closed. An abnormal accentuation of sway or

an actual loss of balance with the eyes closed is a positive result. Visual sense is able to compensate, in part, for a deficiency in conscious recognition of muscle and joint position. Therefore the patient may be able to maintain his balance if he is allowed to open his eyes. Symptoms of ataxia caused by lesions of the cerebellum, on the contrary, are not corrected by visual compensation.

7

TOUCH

Tactile sensations are complex in nature since they involve a blending of light cutaneous contact and variable degrees of pressure, depending upon the intensity of the stimuli. Two different forms of touch sensibility are recognized: simple touch and tactile discrimination. *Simple touch* is concerned with a sense of light touch, light pressure, and a crude sense of tactile localization. Tickling and itching sensations are related to pain sense. *Tactile discrimination* conveys the sense of spatial localization and perception of the size and shape of objects.

The method of testing simple touch is by stroking the skin with a wisp of cotton. Von Frey hairs are used for experimental work. These are a series of fine hairs of graduated stiffness for applying stimuli at calibrated intensity to the skin. Tactile discrimination is tested by having the patient, with eyes closed, describe the location of a touch stimulus on the skin; identify common small objects placed in the patient's hand; determine whether one touch stimulus or two simultaneous stimuli have been applied to the skin; and identify numbers written on the surface of the skin with a blunt object.

PATHWAYS MEDIATING THE SENSATION OF TOUCH

At least three different spinal cord pathways mediate tactile sensation. The *lemniscal pathways* are concerned with the discriminative aspects of touch, including identification of place, contour, and quality of the stimulus. These pathways have been discussed in Chapter 6. The *lateral and ventral spino-thalamic tracts,* components of the *anterolateral system,* subserve touch sensation (Fig. 17). The other component of the anterolateral system, the spinoreticular projections, is concerned with responses to noxious stimuli, as discussed in Chapter 5. Finally, the *lateral cervical system* (spinocervico-thalamic pathway) is thought to mediate touch sensation as well as vibratory and proprioceptive senses.

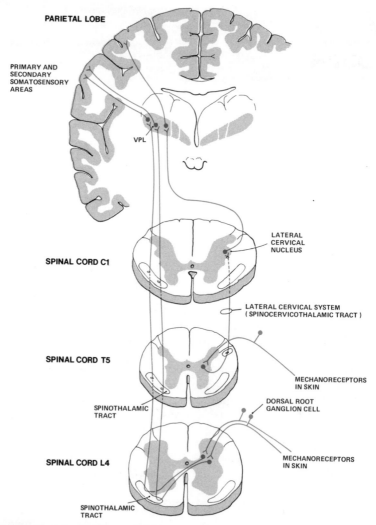

FIGURE 17. The central nervous system pathways mediating tactile sensation except for the lemniscal system. The lateral and ventral components of the lateral spinothalamic tract are shown.

The Lateral and Ventral Spinothalamic Tracts

These pathways were discussed in Chapter 5. Previously, the lateral and ventral components of the spinothalamic tract were thought to subserve different functions, with the lateral spinothalamic tract mediating nociceptive information and the ventral spinothalamic tract mediating tactile sensation. Recent evidence indicates no functional difference between the lateral and ventral components of the spinothalamic tract. Both are capable of mediating nociceptive and tactile sensations.

The Lateral Cervical System

Almost all of the cells of the lateral cervical system are sensitive to light mechanical stimulation of the skin of the ipsilateral side of the body, but a few are activated by noxious stimuli. Peripheral nerve fibers entering this system make synaptic connections in the dorsal horn (laminae III, IV, and V) throughout the length of the spinal cord. Heavily myelinated second-order neurons arise in these laminae and ascend ipsilaterally in the most medial corner of the dorsal lateral funiculus to terminate in the lateral cervical nucleus. This nucleus is located just lateral to the dorsal horn of the first and second cervical segments (see Fig. 17). The axons of these cells cross the spinal cord to join the contralateral medial lemniscus and, with it, terminate within the thalamus. Projections from the thalamus reach the somatic sensory areas of the cerebral cortex. The entire lateral cervical system is very rapidly conducting. The most detailed information about this system now available comes from studies on nonhuman primates and carnivores. The function of this system in human sensory perception is still unknown.

Effect of Sectioning the Pathways Mediating Touch Sensation

Of all types of skin sensibility, simple touch is least likely to be impaired by lesions of the spinal cord. Although tactile discrimination, such as the direction of movement of a cutaneous stimulus, usually is abolished by a lesion of the dorsal column, light touch sensation may be decreased only slightly or not at all on the ipsilateral side by such a lesion. After destruction of the ventral and lateral spinothalamic tracts, pain perception is lost on the opposite side of the body, but light touch generally persists because the dorsal columns also can mediate this function.

8

LESIONS OF THE PERIPHERAL NERVES, SPINAL ROOTS, AND SPINAL CORD

FLACCID PARALYSIS OF MUSCLES: LOWER MOTONEURON LESION

The term "lower motoneuron" is used to designate the anterior horn cells of the spinal cord, which innervate the skeletal muscles of the body, and the motor nerve cells of the brain stem, which innervate muscles supplied by the cranial nerves. Destruction of these neurons (Fig. 18, lesion 4), their axons in ventral nerve roots (Fig. 18, lesion 3), or motor fibers of peripheral nerves (Fig. 18, lesion 1) abolishes both the voluntary and reflex responses of muscles. Besides paralysis, the affected muscles show hypotonia (diminished resistance to passive manipulation of the limbs) and absence of the muscle stretch reflexes. Within a few weeks the fibers of the muscles begin to show *atrophy.* The atrophy of muscle fibers deprived of their motoneurons is more profound than the atrophy that occurs in muscles that are rendered inactive. This is because the anterior horn cells exert a trophic influence on muscle fibers that is essential for maintaining their normal state. Muscles that are undergoing early stages of atrophy display *fibrillations* and *fasciculations.* Fibrillations are fine twitchings of single muscle fibers that generally cannot be seen on clinical examination but can be detected on electromyographic examination. Fasciculations are brief contractions of *motor units,* which can be seen in skeletal muscle through the intact skin. A motor unit consists of a single anterior horn cell; its peripheral

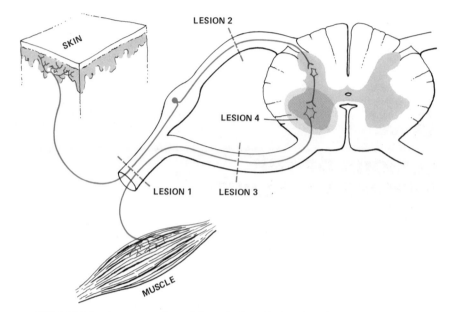

FIGURE 18. A cross section of the spinal cord, dorsal and ventral roots, and peripheral nerve. Lesion 1 affects the peripheral nerve, lesion 2 the dorsal root, lesion 3 the ventral root, and lesion 4 the anterior horn cells.

axon, which commonly branches into several terminal divisions; and each muscle fiber innervated by these branches.

Lesions that damage sensory fibers of the dorsal roots (Fig. 18, lesion 2) or their cell bodies in spinal ganglia also disrupt the stretch reflex pathway (see Fig. 10) and, as a consequence, produce hypotonia and loss of tendon reflexes in the muscles. In this instance the lower motoneurons remain intact, and there is little or no loss of voluntary motor strength. The trophic influence of anterior horn cells is not impaired, and neither muscle atrophy (except that of disuse) nor fasciculations appear.

SPASTIC PARALYSIS OF MUSCLES: UPPER MOTONEURON LESION

The term "upper motoneuron" is used to describe nerve cell bodies that originate in central nervous system structures, such as the cerebral cortex and brain stem, and send their axons into the spinal cord where they make contact, directly or indirectly, with anterior horn cells. Examples of upper motoneuron pathways include the corticospinal, reticulospinal, vestibulospinal, and rubrospinal tracts.

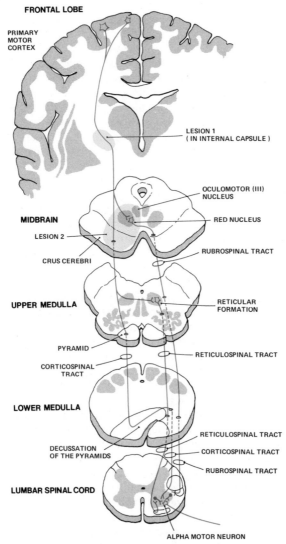

FRONTAL LOBE

PRIMARY MOTOR CORTEX

LESION 1
(IN INTERNAL CAPSULE)

OCULOMOTOR (III) NUCLEUS

MIDBRAIN

RED NUCLEUS

LESION 2

RUBROSPINAL TRACT

CRUS CEREBRI

UPPER MEDULLA

RETICULAR FORMATION

PYRAMID

RETICULOSPINAL TRACT

CORTICOSPINAL TRACT

LOWER MEDULLA

RETICULOSPINAL TRACT

DECUSSATION OF THE PYRAMIDS

CORTICOSPINAL TRACT

RUBROSPINAL TRACT

LUMBAR SPINAL CORD

ALPHA MOTOR NEURON

FIGURE 19. Several of the major motor pathways of the central nervous system. Lesion 1 affects the internal capsule and causes a contralateral hemiplegia affecting the lower portion of the face and the arm and leg. Lesion 2 causes an ipsilateral cranial nerve disorder (loss of function of the third cranial nerve) and a contralateral hemiplegia affecting the lower portion of the face and the arm and leg.

A lesion in the posterior limb of the internal capsule (Fig. 19, lesion 1) disrupts the influence of the cerebral cortex upon anterior horn cells on the contralateral side of the body. The corticospinal tract is only one of many pathways involved in such a lesion since the lesion also interrupts connections between the cerebral cortex and the origin of the rubrospinal and reticulospinal pathways. Immediately following such a lesion, the patient develops paralysis of the face, arm, and leg *(hemiplegia)* of the opposite side of the body with hypotonia and depression of the muscle stretch reflexes. After an interval that varies from a few days to a few weeks, stretch reflexes return in these muscles and then progress to become more active than normal. Hypertonia develops, as shown by fixed postures of the limbs and increased resistance to passive manipulation of the limbs. As the examiner manipulates the limbs, the resistance is most marked in the flexor muscles of the arm and the extensor muscles of the leg. This resistance is strong at the beginning of the movement but gives way in a "clasp-knife" fashion as the movement is continued. The muscle stretch reflexes are hyperactive and occasionally may show *clonus,* a sustained series of rhythmic jerks, as a tendon is maintained in extension by the examiner. Muscles showing these signs of hyperreflexia are said to be spastic or to show spasticity. Other conditions may produce hypertonic muscles, but they have distinguishing features that differentiate them from the spasticity associated with internal capsule lesions. Some examples of these are decerebrate rigidity, dystonia, parkinsonian rigidity, and myotonia. In addition to spastic weakness with hyperreflexia, internal capsule lesions result in the Babinski sign. This reflex response is described in the next section.

The pyramidal tract consists of nerve cell bodies arising in the cerebral cortex with axons coursing through the pyramidal tract in the medulla and terminating on anterior horn cells or interneurons in the spinal cord. The pyramidal tract is also termed the corticospinal tract. In the older literature, signs of upper motoneuron disease (e.g., spastic paralysis, increased muscle stretch reflexes, clonus, Babinski sign, "clasp-knife" response to passive movements, and lack of muscle atrophy except for disuse atrophy) have been attributed to pyramidal (corticospinal) tract lesions. The corticospinal tract, through its termination on lower motoneurons, was thought previously to have the capacity of restricting the activity of the stretch reflex. Spasticity was explained as the enhancement (release) of stretch reflexes from the inhibitory influence of the corticospinal tract. There are very few case reports of humans with lesions restricted to the pyramidal tract, and it is debatable whether a lesion in this site will produce signs of the upper motoneuron syndrome. In addition, activity of the stretch reflex is regulated by the balanced effects of all of the fiber tracts descending to the spinal cord from the brain stem as well as the corticospinal tract. Some of these descending systems have inhibitory effects, and others have facilitatory effects. Spasticity and increased deep tendon reflexes can result from a net reduction of inhibitory influences upon alpha and gamma motoneurons. Hypersensitive gamma fibers can stimulate muscle spindles to a higher rate of discharge, resulting in enhanced responses to muscle stretch. Hypersensitive alpha motoneurons can react excessively to proprioceptive input from muscle stretch receptors. It is not yet clear whether the responses of both gamma and alpha motoneurons are enhanced in spasticity. The bulk of evidence suggests that hyperactive alpha motoneurons account for the abnormalities.

It is important to bear in mind that the symptoms listed for corticospinal tract lesions occur because other descending pathways tend to be involved as well. The only neurologic sign that clearly can be attributed to lesions of the corticospinal tract is the Babinski sign. A corticospinal tract lesion rostral to the level of the pyramidal decussation gives rise to contralateral spasticity, muscle weakness, and the Babinski sign. A lesion of this tract caudal to the level of the pyramidal decussation causes these signs on the ipsilateral side of the body.

The effects of lower motoneuron lesions are limited to the muscles that they innervate, but a small lesion that interrupts the corticospinal tract removes voluntary motor control from the whole sector of the body that lies downstream from the level of the injury. Thus a lesion of the posterior limb of the internal capsule (see Fig. 19, lesion 1) causes paralysis of the contralateral face, arm, and leg. Involvement of the face is limited to the lower portions of the face because the muscles in the upper portions are innervated by lower motoneurons that receive their innervation from both cerebral hemispheres. A lesion on one side of the brain stem commonly affects one of the cranial nerves (the third nerve in the instance of lesion 2 in Figure 19), and thus the patient will have loss of function of a cranial nerve on the side ipsilateral to the lesion with a hemiplegia on the contralateral side.

Paralysis affecting the arm and leg of one side of the body is termed *hemiplegia. Paraplegia* is paralysis of both legs, as, for example, after a transverse lesion of the spinal cord that destroys the upper motoneurons of both sides of the cord. Paralysis of a single extremity is *monoplegia,* and one that includes all four extremities is *quadriplegia.* Lesions that impair function but are not severe enough to cause total paralysis produce weakness that is clinically designated as *paresis.*

OTHER REFLEXES ASSOCIATED WITH LESIONS OF THE MOTOR PATHWAY

Certain reflexes that are not elicited in normal individuals may be present after injuries of the corticospinal tract. The *Babinski sign* is an abnormal reflex obtained by stroking the plantar surface of the outer border of the foot with a blunt point. The normal response is plantar flexion of the great toe, but if the Babinski sign is present there is a slow dorsiflexion of the great toe, at times accompanied by fanning of the other toes. When it is found, the Babinski sign is a strong indication of a disorder of the corticospinal tract. Many similar pathologic reflexes have been described. *Hoff-*

mann's sign is sought by flicking the nail of the patient's middle finger. When the sign is present there is prompt adduction of the thumb and flexion of the index finger. Hoffmann's sign is commonly associated with injury of the pyramidal tract, but it occurs occasionally in normal persons.

Superficial reflexes, which normally are obtained by stroking certain areas of the skin, may be absent if the corticospinal tract is injured. If the skin of the abdominal wall is scratched gently, the abdominal musculature contracts locally, causing the umbilicus to deviate momentarily in the direction of the stimulus. Stroking the upper, inner aspect of the thigh normally causes reflex contraction of the cremaster muscle with elevation of the testicle on the stimulated side. Loss of these *abdominal* or *cremasteric* reflexes confirms the presence of a corticospinal tract lesion, but absence of these reflexes bilaterally in an otherwise normal individual may have no significance.

LESIONS OF PERIPHERAL NERVES

Injury of an individual peripheral nerve (see Fig. 18, lesion 1) is followed by paralysis of muscles and loss of sensation limited to those muscles and skin areas supplied by the nerve distal to the lesion. The paralyzed muscles are flaccid and gradually undergo severe atrophy. All forms of sensation, including proprioception, are lost. Recognition of peripheral nerve lesions is based on knowledge of the course and distribution of such nerves.

In polyneuritis there is partial destruction of various peripheral nerves. The distribution of the lesions is frequently bilateral, and the effects are usually more prominent in the distal parts of the extremities. Muscular weakness and atrophy accompanied by sensory loss in the distal portions of the extremities (often in a "glove and stocking" distribution) are characteristic of this disorder.

LESIONS OF THE POSTERIOR ROOTS

Tabes dorsalis is a form of neurosyphilis that causes bilateral degeneration of dorsal nerve roots and of the posterior funiculi secondarily, particularly in the lower segments of the spinal cord. Irritation of nerve root fibers is thought to account for *paresthesias* (sensations of numbness and tingling) and intermittent attacks of sharp pain that characteristically appear early in the course of the disease. As destruction progresses there is diminished sensitivity to pain with the result that the skin, bone, and joints can be severely damaged without the patient's knowledge. Interruption of the stretch reflex arcs in the posterior roots leads to loss of the patellar reflexes (muscle stretch reflexes elicited from the quadriceps) and ankle jerks (muscle stretch reflexes elicited from the gastrocnemius). There is severe impairment both of position sense and of vibratory sense. A positive Romberg sign is present. This sign is demonstrated by having the patient stand with feet together and eyes open. If the patient is steady with eyes open, he is asked to close his eyes. Loss of balance with the eyes closed constitutes a positive Romberg sign. This occurs because visual cues about the patient's position in space compensate for the loss of proprioceptive input from the legs. The patient walks with legs apart, head bent forward, eyes fixed on the ground, elevating the legs excessively and slapping the feet down.

LESIONS OF THE ANTERIOR HORNS

Poliomyelitis, or infantile paralysis, is caused by a virus that invades anterior horn cells, particularly in the cervical and lumbar enlargements of the spinal cord, often damaging them in large numbers. The extent of the muscle paralysis and the muscle groups affected vary, depending on the distribution of motor cells that fail to recover. Paralyzed muscles are flaccid, and their reflexes are usually absent. Atrophy develops after several weeks, and paralyzed muscles ultimately may be replaced by connective and adipose tissue. Severe paralysis is likely to result in extensive deformities. Characteristically, poliomyelitis is a patchy and asymmetric process.

LESIONS OF THE CENTRAL GRAY MATTER

In *syringomyelia* there is progressive cavitation around or near the central canal of the spinal cord, most commonly in the region of the cervical enlargement. A lesion in this position interrupts the lateral spinothalamic fibers that pass ventral to the central canal as they cross from one side to the other (Fig. 20A, lesion enclosed by dotted line). Since these fibers conduct pain and temperature impulses from dermatomes on both sides of the body, the result is loss of pain and temperature sensibility with a segmental distribution in the upper extremities on both sides. Because the spinothalamic tracts themselves remain intact, there is no sensory impairment in the lower extremities. Proprioception and the sense of simple touch are spared in the affected dermatomes of the arms. A condition such as this, in which one type of skin sense is lost and others preserved, is referred to as *sensory dissociation.* In later stages of the disease, degeneration often extends to the anterior gray horns (Fig. 20A, shaded area) and causes paralysis with atrophy of muscles innervated by the segments involved. Signs of upper motoneuron disease may appear in the lower extremities as a result of compression of the lateral corticospinal tracts by the cystic cavity.

LESIONS INVOLVING BOTH THE ANTERIOR HORNS AND THE PYRAMIDAL TRACTS

Amyotrophic lateral sclerosis is a progressive, fatal disease of unknown cause characterized by destruction of motor cells in the anterior gray horns of the spinal cord together with degeneration of the pyramidal tracts bilaterally. Sensory changes usually do not occur. Weakness and atrophy are noted in some muscles, with spasticity and hyperreflexia in others. The effects may be somewhat irregular in distribution, depending on individual variations in the pattern of the lesions in the spinal cord. The classic form of this disease starts with weakness, atrophy, and fasciculations of the muscles of the hands and arms, followed later by spastic paralysis of the limbs. In some cases, motor nuclei of the lower cranial nerves undergo degeneration.

LESIONS INVOLVING POSTERIOR AND LATERAL FUNICULI

Subacute combined degeneration is a disease of the spinal cord most often seen in pernicious anemia but sometimes occurring with other types of anemia or nutritional disturbances. The dorsal columns and the lateral columns of the spinal cord undergo degeneration, but the gray matter ordinarily is not affected. Injury of the dorsal columns is accompanied by loss of position sense in the lower extremities, impairment of ability to recognize vibration over the legs, and a positive Romberg sign. Motor weakness in the legs with spasticity, hyperactive tendon reflexes, and bilateral Babinski signs indicate degeneration of the upper motoneuron projections in the lateral columns.

THROMBOSIS OF THE ANTERIOR SPINAL ARTERY

The anterior spinal artery runs in the anterior median sulcus and sends terminal branches to supply the ventral and lateral funiculi and most of the gray matter of the spinal cord. The anterior horns, the lateral spinothalamic tracts, and the pyramidal tracts are included in its territory, but the dorsal funiculi and posterior part of the dorsal horns are supplied independently by a pair of posterior spinal arteries. Thrombosis of the anterior spinal artery in the cervical region of the cord produces atrophy, fasciculations, and flaccid paralysis at the level of the lesion due to destruction of anterior horn cells. There will also be spastic paraplegia from bilateral corticospinal tract involvement and, usually, loss of pain and temperature sense below the lesion due to bilateral spinothalamic tract damage. The onset of symptoms is abrupt and is often accompanied by severe pain.

HEMISECTION OF THE SPINAL CORD

Lateral hemisection of the spinal cord (as, for example, from a bullet or knife wound) produces the *Brown-Séquard syndrome* (Fig. 20B). The specific effects in the patient with a chronic lesion and the injured structures that account for them are summarized below.

Effects from Injury to Fiber Tracts

On the side of the lesion, effects from injury to the fiber tracts include:

1. Lateral column damage, involving paralysis below the injury with spasticity, hyperactive reflexes, clonus, loss of superficial reflexes, and the Babinski sign.

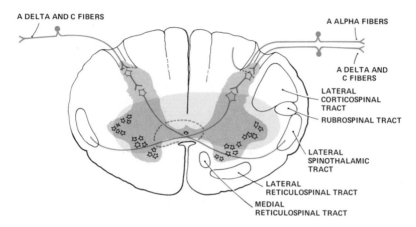

A. Syringomyelia

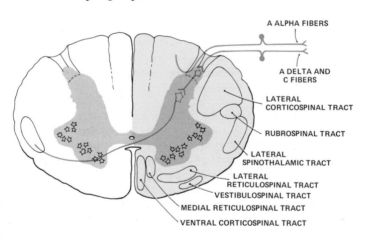

B. Brown-Séquard Lesion

FIGURE 20. *A.* A cross section of the spinal cord showing the pathways interrupted by a cavitating lesion of syringomyelia of small size *(dotted line)* and larger size *(shaded area). B.* A cross section of the spinal cord showing the pathways interrupted by a hemisection of the cord (Brown-Séquard lesion).

2. Dorsal column damage, involving loss of position sense, vibratory sense, and tactile discrimination below the injury. Because of the paralysis, ataxia which might otherwise occur cannot be demonstrated readily.

Damage to the anterolateral system involves loss of the sensations of pain and temperature on the side opposite the lesion beginning one or two dermatomes below the injury.

Effects from Injury to Local Cord Segments and Nerve Roots

Besides the effects produced by interrupting the long ascending and descending tracts of the spinal cord, symptoms are likely from damage to dorsal and ventral nerve roots at the level of the injury. These symptoms occur on the side of the lesion, and when present, they are of great value in localizing the individual cord segments involved.

1. Irritation of fibers in the dorsal root zone: paresthesias or radicular pain in a band over the affected dermatomes.
2. Destruction of dorsal roots: a band of anesthesia over the dermatome supplied by the involved roots.
3. Destruction of ventral roots: flaccid paralysis affecting only those muscles innervated by fibers that have been destroyed.

Few lesions are precisely localized to one lateral half of the spinal cord. More often they involve one sector of the cord and produce a partial, or incomplete, Brown-Séquard syndrome. The particular symptoms and signs in each case are determined by the position and extent of the lesion.

TUMORS OF THE SPINAL CORD

Tumors that arise within the vertebral canal but outside the spinal cord (extramedullary tumors) gradually impinge on the cord as they enlarge. Compression of nerve roots often occurs first and accounts for pain distributed over the dermatomes supplied by these roots. This is followed by gradual involvement of the tracts within the spinal cord until a Brown-Séquard syndrome, or some modification of it, is reached. The order of appearance of symptoms may furnish a clue to the site of the tumor. For example, loss of pain and temperature sensibility involving all segments below a certain level on the left side followed by spastic paralysis on the right implies that the tumor has arisen from the ventrolateral region of the cord on the right side. Loss of proprioception sense on the right side followed by an extension of the proprioceptive deficit to the left side and the development of spastic paralysis on the right indicates that the tumor is compressing the spinal cord from the dorsomedial region on the right side.

Injuries to nerve fibers in the spinal cord vary in degree. Some are sufficient to prevent conduction of nerve impulses without causing irreversible fiber degeneration. The pressure of tumors, herniated intervertebral disks, blood clots, or the swelling and edema of wounds may produce spinal cord symptoms that are later alleviated by treatment. The prospect of recovery depends on the severity of the pressure and its duration.

DEGENERATIVE CHANGES IN NERVE CELLS

When a fiber is transected or permanently destroyed, the part that has been separated from the nerve cell body degenerates completely and, in the process, loses its myelin sheath. Degenerated fibers can be studied histologically by obtaining a series of microscopic sections, staining them appropriately, and reconstructing the course of the fibers. The Weigert and Weil methods employ a modified hematoxylin stain that stains normal myelin dark blue or black. An unstained area appearing in the position normally occupied by a fiber tract indicates degeneration, although degenerating fibers are not visible. The Marchi method utilizes impregnation of the sections with osmium tetroxide to blacken degenerating nerve fibers while leaving normal myelinated fibers unstained. The test is effective only if osmium tetroxide is applied at a particular stage of the degenerative process when myelin is partly, but not completely, decomposed (generally 6 to 12 days after injury). For this reason the Marchi method is rarely suitable for use with human postmortem material but has been used extensively in experimental work. The *Nauta method* and its modifications (*Nauta-Gygax* and *Fink-Heimer*) are invaluable techniques in tracing degenerating axons. These silver nitrate impregnation techniques have a tremendous advantage over the Marchi method in that the degenerating axon (including its terminal processes, telodendria, and boutons), rather than the myelin sheath, is impregnated.

Besides causing permanent destruction of the disconnected portion, severing a cell's axon has a harmful effect on the nerve cell body itself. For several weeks after the injury, the Nissl bodies (chromophilic substance) of the cell undergo *chromatolysis,* a process in which extranuclear granules of RNA lose their staining characteristics and seem to dissolve in the surrounding cytoplasm. Some of the affected cells disintegrate, but others recover with restoration of Nissl substance. As Nissl himself realized, this retrograde chromatolytic reaction furnishes a means of determining the cells of origin for fibers. Some weeks following a lesion placed in the central nervous system of an experimental animal serial sections stained for Nissl substance with a basic aniline dye may reveal specific areas of chromatolysis.

REGENERATION OF NERVE FIBERS

A completely severed peripheral nerve has some capacity to repair itself. *Schwann* (neurolemma) cells derived from the myelin of the central end of the nerve stump proliferate and attempt to bridge the gap with the distal end of the nerve. The axis cylinders in the central end of the cut nerve divide longitudinally and soon begin to sprout out of the end of the nerve. Many sprouting axons go astray in random directions, but some of them cross the gap and enter neurilemmal tubes leading to the peripheral endings. Their rate of growth is normally 1 to 2 mm per day. Chance apparently determines whether a regenerating motor fiber enters a neurilemmal tube leading to a motor or to a sensory terminal. If suitably matched, connections with a motor end-plate can be re-established and function restored. Fibers of the brain and of the spinal cord, however, do not regenerate effectively.

9

THE BRAIN STEM: MEDULLA, PONS, AND MIDBRAIN

MEDULLA

The medulla (medulla oblongata, or bulb) is the most caudal part of the brain stem. It is continuous with the spinal cord at the foramen magnum and extends rostrally for 2.5 cm to the caudal border of the pons. The central canal of the spinal cord continues through the caudal half of the medulla and then, at a point called the *obex*, flares open into the wide cavity of the fourth ventricle. The rostral part of the medulla thus occupies the floor of the fourth ventricle. The roof of the ventricle is formed by the tela choroidea and *choroid plexus*, a thin sheet of ependyma and pia mater with blood vessels between them.

External Markings of the Medulla

ANTERIOR (VENTRAL) ASPECT. The *pyramids*, which contain the pyramidal *(corticospinal)* tracts, form two longitudinal ridges on either side of the ventral median fissure (Fig. 21). Their decussation can be seen obliterating the fissure at the extreme caudal end of the medulla.

LATERAL ASPECT. Two longitudinal grooves are present, the ventrolateral sulcus and the dorsolateral sulcus (Fig. 22). The ventrolateral sulcus extends along the lateral border of the pyramid, and from this groove exit

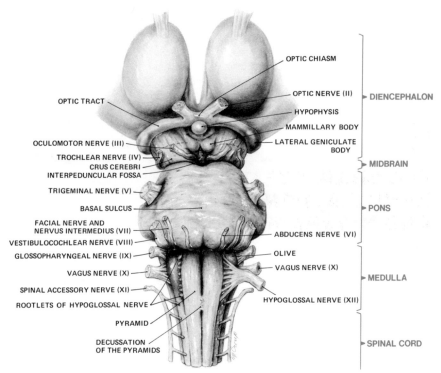

FIGURE 21. The ventral surface of the human brain stem and diencephalon.

the rootlets of the hypoglossal nerve (n. XII). Radicles of the bulbar accessory nerve (n. XI), vagus nerve (n. X), and glossopharyngeal nerve (n. IX) are attached in line along the dorsolateral sulcus. The spinal portion of the accessory nerve (n. XI) arises from the gray matter of spinal cord segments C-2 to C-5. Its rootlets exit through the lateral funiculus of the cord, join, and ascend along the lateral surface of the medulla. The prominent oval swelling of the lateral area of the medulla between the ventrolateral and dorsolateral sulci is the *olive* (see Figs. 21 and 22). This marks the site of the inferior olivary nuclear complex inside the medulla.

POSTERIOR (DORSAL) ASPECT. Figures 21, 22, and 23 represent specimens of the brain stem from which the overlying cerebellum and the ependymal roof of the fourth ventricle have been removed. The fasciculus gracilis and the fasciculus cuneatus are visible as low ridges. The sites of termination of these two tracts in the nucleus gracilis and the nucleus cuneatus are marked by small eminences named, respectively, the *clava* and the *cuneate tubercle*. The fibers from the nuclei gracilis and cuneatus descend into the tegmentum of the brain stem; thus this area "opens up," exposing the floor of the fourth ventricle rostral to the obex. Two pairs of small swellings can be seen in the floor of the ventricle. Their tapering

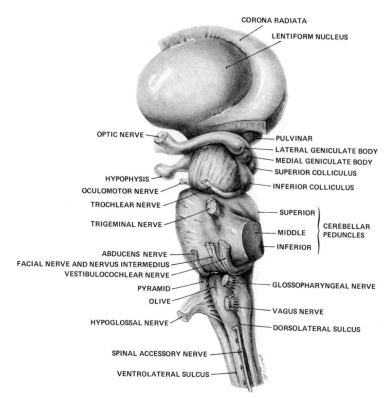

CORONA RADIATA
LENTIFORM NUCLEUS

OPTIC NERVE
PULVINAR
LATERAL GENICULATE BODY
MEDIAL GENICULATE BODY
HYPOPHYSIS
SUPERIOR COLLICULUS
OCULOMOTOR NERVE
INFERIOR COLLICULUS
TROCHLEAR NERVE
TRIGEMINAL NERVE
SUPERIOR
MIDDLE
INFERIOR
CEREBELLAR PEDUNCLES
ABDUCENS NERVE
FACIAL NERVE AND NERVUS INTERMEDIUS
VESTIBULOCOCHLEAR NERVE
PYRAMID
OLIVE
GLOSSOPHARYNGEAL NERVE
HYPOGLOSSAL NERVE
VAGUS NERVE
SPINAL ACCESSORY NERVE
DORSOLATERAL SULCUS
VENTROLATERAL SULCUS

FIGURE 22. The lateral surface of the human brain stem, lentiform nucleus, and corona radiata.

margins point caudally and gradually meet the groove of the medial sulcus in a configuration named the *calamus scriptorius* from its resemblance to the point of a pen. The lateral ridges of the calamus constitute the *vagal trigone;* the medial ridges are the *hypoglossal trigone.* These trigones are bulges that indicate the locations of underlying nuclei, the dorsal motor nucleus of the vagus and the hypoglossal nucleus respectively. The *striae medullares of the fourth ventricle* are ridges formed by fibers passing toward the cerebellum. Laterally these fibers mark the location of the *lateral recesses.* At these sites, openings from the fourth ventricle allow CSF to pass from the ventricular system into the subarachnoid space.

Internal Structures of the Medulla
Some of the long fiber tracts of the spinal cord (e.g., spinothalamic tracts) pass directly through the medulla without any major changes in their relative positions, but both the corticospinal fibers and the dorsal columns of the spinal cord undergo shifts that radically change the arrangement of the gray and white matter in the medulla as compared to the cord.

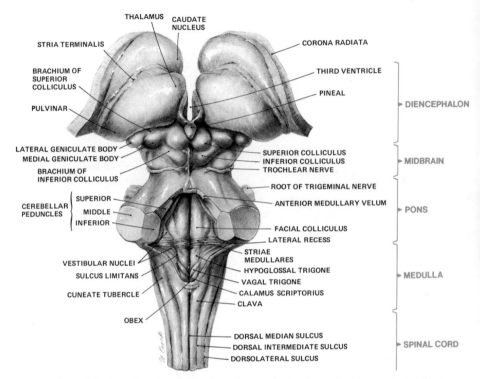

FIGURE 23. The dorsal surface of the human brain stem, diencephalon, caudate nucleus, and corona radiata. The cerebellum has been removed by cutting through the peduncles.

Figures 24 through 30 are drawings of histologic sections of the human brain stem. These thin slices of tissue were cut perpendicular to the long axis of the brain stem and stained with the Weigert method, in which chemicals in the stain bind to components of myelin. Thus the dark areas on these cross sections represent myelinated fibers, and the light areas represent areas free of such fibers, which are usually filled with neuron cell bodies forming the various nuclei of the brain stem.

CAUDAL HALF OF THE MEDULLA. A *central gray area* surrounds the central canal and merges at its perimeter with a zone containing a network of fibers and cells known as the *reticular formation*. The reticular formation extends through the medulla, pons, and midbrain. It is an area that contains nuclear groups carrying out vital functions, such as the control of blood pressure and respiration.

The corticospinal tracts descend through the most anterior part of the medulla in the pyramids and, at the caudal end of the medulla, most of these fibers cross in a prominent decussation that brings them to the lateral

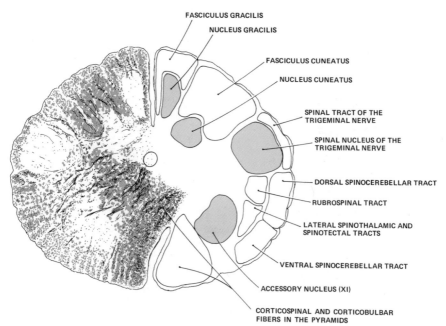

FASCICULUS GRACILIS
NUCLEUS GRACILIS
FASCICULUS CUNEATUS
NUCLEUS CUNEATUS
SPINAL TRACT OF THE TRIGEMINAL NERVE
SPINAL NUCLEUS OF THE TRIGEMINAL NERVE
DORSAL SPINOCEREBELLAR TRACT
RUBROSPINAL TRACT
LATERAL SPINOTHALAMIC AND SPINOTECTAL TRACTS
VENTRAL SPINOCEREBELLAR TRACT
ACCESSORY NUCLEUS (XI)
CORTICOSPINAL AND CORTICOBULBAR FIBERS IN THE PYRAMIDS

FIGURE 24. Cross section of the lowest level of the medulla, through the decussation of the pyramids. The left side of the diagram represents the general appearance of this level in a myelin-stained histologic preparation. On the right side the major tracts *(open)* and nuclei *(color)* are outlined and labeled.

position they maintain in the spinal cord (Fig. 24). On the posterior side the fasciculi gracilis and cuneatus remain present, but the nuclei in which their fibers terminate have appeared. Axons of the cells in these nuclei take a downward, arched course, forming the *internal arcuate fibers* that cross the midline as the *decussation* of the *medial lemniscus* (Fig. 25). Lateral to the rostral part of the cuneate nucleus the *accessory cuneate nucleus* appears. Cells in this nucleus do not contribute to the medial lemniscus, but ascend laterally into the inferior cerebellar peduncle as the cuneocerebellar tract (see Fig. 15). In the posterolateral region a clear nuclear area, capped by a peripheral zone of fine fibers, represents the *spinal tract* and *spinal nucleus of the trigeminal nerve.* The latter structures reach the lower medulla by descending from the pontine region.

ROSTRAL HALF OF THE MEDULLA. The principal nucleus of the *inferior olivary nuclear complex,* a prominent structure in the anterolateral region, resembles a crinkled sac with an opening directed toward the midline (Fig. 26). Many of its efferent fibers cross the midline and stream toward the posterolateral corner of the medulla to join spinocerebellar fibers in the thick *inferior cerebellar peduncle.*

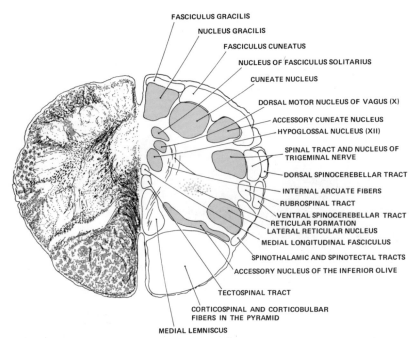

FASCICULUS GRACILIS
NUCLEUS GRACILIS
FASCICULUS CUNEATUS
NUCLEUS OF FASCICULUS SOLITARIUS
CUNEATE NUCLEUS
DORSAL MOTOR NUCLEUS OF VAGUS (X)
ACCESSORY CUNEATE NUCLEUS
HYPOGLOSSAL NUCLEUS (XII)
SPINAL TRACT AND NUCLEUS OF TRIGEMINAL NERVE
DORSAL SPINOCEREBELLAR TRACT
INTERNAL ARCUATE FIBERS
RUBROSPINAL TRACT
VENTRAL SPINOCEREBELLAR TRACT
RETICULAR FORMATION
LATERAL RETICULAR NUCLEUS
MEDIAL LONGITUDINAL FASCICULUS
SPINOTHALAMIC AND SPINOTECTAL TRACTS
ACCESSORY NUCLEUS OF THE INFERIOR OLIVE
TECTOSPINAL TRACT
CORTICOSPINAL AND CORTICOBULBAR FIBERS IN THE PYRAMID
MEDIAL LEMNISCUS

FIGURE 25. Cross section of the lower medulla at the level of the decussation of the internal arcuate fibers forming the medial lemniscus.

Several distinct cellular areas (symmetrically paired) occupy the posterior part of the medulla close to the floor of the ventricle. Since they extend longitudinally through the upper medulla, they represent nuclear columns. The *nucleus of the hypoglossal nerve* (n. XII) is nearest the midline. Fibers of this nerve pass anterior to emerge between the pyramid and the olive. The hypoglossal nerve innervates the striated muscles of the tongue. The *dorsal motor nucleus of the vagus nerve* (n. X) lies at the side of the hypoglossal nucleus and contains neurons that form an important part of the parasympathetic division of the autonomic nervous system. The most lateral nuclear column, separated from the motor nuclei by the sulcus limitans, contains the medial and inferior *vestibular nuclei,* which receive afferent fibers from the vestibular division of the vestibulocochlear nerve (n. VIII). This nerve brings information to the brain concerning position and movement of the head in space.

The *nucleus ambiguus,* seen indistinctly in Weigert-stained preparations, is located in the anterolateral part of the reticular formation. Its fibers course posteromedially at first, but they arch back and leave the medulla anterior to the inferior cerebellar peduncle with fibers of the glossopharyngeal (n. IX), vagus (n. X), and bulbar accessory (n. XI) nerves. These nerve fibers control the branchiomeric muscles of the pharynx and larynx and thus control swallowing and vocalization. An isolated bundle of longitudinal

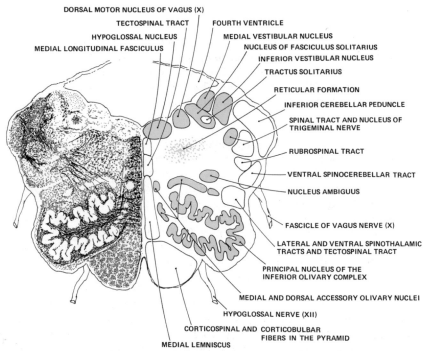

DORSAL MOTOR NUCLEUS OF VAGUS (X)
TECTOSPINAL TRACT
HYPOGLOSSAL NUCLEUS
MEDIAL LONGITUDINAL FASCICULUS
FOURTH VENTRICLE
MEDIAL VESTIBULAR NUCLEUS
NUCLEUS OF FASCICULUS SOLITARIUS
INFERIOR VESTIBULAR NUCLEUS
TRACTUS SOLITARIUS
RETICULAR FORMATION
INFERIOR CEREBELLAR PEDUNCLE
SPINAL TRACT AND NUCLEUS OF TRIGEMINAL NERVE
RUBROSPINAL TRACT
VENTRAL SPINOCEREBELLAR TRACT
NUCLEUS AMBIGUUS
FASCICLE OF VAGUS NERVE (X)
LATERAL AND VENTRAL SPINOTHALAMIC TRACTS AND TECTOSPINAL TRACT
PRINCIPAL NUCLEUS OF THE INFERIOR OLIVARY COMPLEX
MEDIAL AND DORSAL ACCESSORY OLIVARY NUCLEI
HYPOGLOSSAL NERVE (XII)
CORTICOSPINAL AND CORTICOBULBAR FIBERS IN THE PYRAMID
MEDIAL LEMNISCUS

FIGURE 26. Cross section of the upper medulla.

fibers accompanied by a small nucleus appears in the posterior part of the reticular formation. It is known as the *solitary tract* and is made up of afferent root fibers from the facial, glossopharyngeal, and vagus nerves. The cells of the *nucleus of the solitary tract* surround the tract and receive fibers from the tract that carry information about taste and visceral sensations. The spinal tract and nucleus of V continue rostrally in a lateral position and somewhat ventral to the other nuclei surrounding the ventricle.

The anterolateral fiber system from the spinal cord (including the spinothalamic tracts) is adjacent to the nucleus ambiguus on its anterolateral side. Two large bands of fibers lie vertically at either side of the midline. The extreme posterior portion of each band contains the *medial longitudinal fasciculus (MLF)*, a structure that extends from the cervical spinal cord to the midbrain. At this level in the medulla it contains several descending pathways, including the *medial vestibulospinal, tectospinal, interstitiospinal,* and some of the *pontine reticulospinal tracts*. The *medial lemniscus* comprises the remainder and largest portion of this vertical band.

PONS

The pons is a large mass rostral to the medulla. The cerebral peduncles pass into it from above and the pyramids emerge from its caudal margin.

External Markings of the Pons

ANTERIOR ASPECT. This surface is entirely occupied by a band of thick, transverse fibers, which constitutes the pons proper (see Fig. 21). A shallow furrow (the basal sulcus) extends along the midline, coinciding with the course of the basilar artery. The *abducens nerves* (n. VI) take exit in the inferior pontine sulcus at the caudal border of the pons close to the pyramids.

LATERAL ASPECT. The transverse fibers of the pons are funneled into compact lateral bundles—the *middle cerebellar peduncles* (brachia pontis)—that attach the pons to the overlying cerebellum (see Fig. 22). The triangular space formed between the caudal border of the middle cerebellar peduncle, the adjoining part of the cerebellum, and the upper part of the medulla constitutes the cerebellopontine angle. The *facial nerve* (n. VII) and the *vestibulocochlear nerve* (n. VIII) are attached to the brain stem in this niche. The *trigeminal nerve* (n. V), one of the largest of the cranial nerves, penetrates the brachium pontis near the middle of the lateral surface of the pons.

POSTERIOR ASPECT. The posterior surface of the pons forms the rostral floor of the fourth ventricle (see Fig. 23). It is a triangular area with its widest point at the pontomedullary junction where the lateral recesses of the ventricle are situated. Faint, transverse striations observed in this region are named the *striae medullares.* They are formed by arcuatocerebellar fibers and are totally unrelated to the acoustic system. Rostral to the striae medullares in the floor of the ventricle is the *facial colliculus.* This colliculus ("little hill") is formed by the abducens nucleus (n. VI) and the fibers of the facial nerve (n. VII) that cross over the nucleus of VI (Fig. 27). The two bands which course along the sides of the triangular space are the *superior cerebellar peduncles* (brachia conjunctiva). The *anterior medullary* velum is a thin layer of tissue completing the roof of the ventricle.

Internal Structure of the Pons

Internal examination of the pons reveals two evident subdivisions: a posterior portion known as the *tegmentum* and an anterior part called the *basilar portion.* In this region of the brain stem, the roof portion, overlying the cavity of the ventricle, has become expanded and specialized to form the cerebellum.

CAUDAL PORTION. The corticospinal tracts are located centrally in the basilar portion. The gray matter that surrounds them contains the cells of the *pontine nuclei.* Transverse pontine fibers (pontocerebellar tract) crossing from one side to the other posterior and anterior to the corticospinal tracts are the axons of cell bodies in the pontine nuclei. They form the

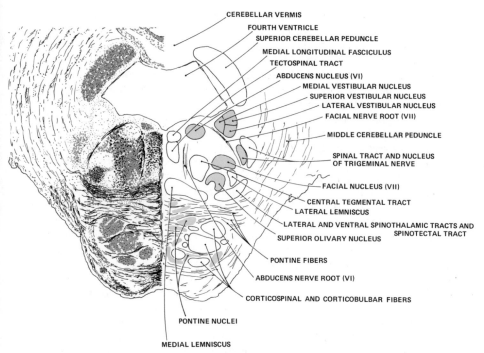

CEREBELLAR VERMIS
FOURTH VENTRICLE
SUPERIOR CEREBELLAR PEDUNCLE
MEDIAL LONGITUDINAL FASCICULUS
TECTOSPINAL TRACT
ABDUCENS NUCLEUS (VI)
MEDIAL VESTIBULAR NUCLEUS
SUPERIOR VESTIBULAR NUCLEUS
LATERAL VESTIBULAR NUCLEUS
FACIAL NERVE ROOT (VII)
MIDDLE CEREBELLAR PEDUNCLE
SPINAL TRACT AND NUCLEUS OF TRIGEMINAL NERVE
FACIAL NUCLEUS (VII)
CENTRAL TEGMENTAL TRACT
LATERAL LEMNISCUS
LATERAL AND VENTRAL SPINOTHALAMIC TRACTS AND SPINOTECTAL TRACT
SUPERIOR OLIVARY NUCLEUS
PONTINE FIBERS
ABDUCENS NERVE ROOT (VI)
CORTICOSPINAL AND CORTICOBULBAR FIBERS
PONTINE NUCLEI
MEDIAL LEMNISCUS

FIGURE 27. Cross section of the pons at the level of the nuclei of cranial nerves VI and VII.

middle cerebellar peduncle and pass to the cortex of the cerebellum. The pontine nuclei receive input from the cerebrum, and their projections to the cerebellum constitute a major route by which the cerebral cortex communicates with the cerebellar cortex.

The *medial lemniscus* is seen as an ellipsoid bundle of fibers. In the medulla the long axis of this ellipse is oriented in the anterior-posterior axis. In the pons these fibers have shifted, and the long axis of the ellipse now extends transversely and contacts the basilar portion of the pons. The *medial longitudinal fasciculus* (MLF) retains its position near the midline in the floor of the fourth ventricle. At this level of the pons, the main ascending fibers in the MLF arise from the vestibular nuclei and project primarily to the nuclei supplying the extraocular muscles. The *interstitiospinal, pontine reticulospinal, tectospinal,* and *tectobulbar tracts* are partially intermingled with the MLF.

The *trapezoid body* (an auditory relay structure) is a prominent band of decussating fibers intermingled with small nuclear groups in the anterior part of the tegmentum. Its fibers interlace at right angles with those of the medial lemniscus. The *superior olive* is a small oval nucleus that lies lateral and slightly posterior to the trapezoid body. It, too, is a structure belonging to the auditory system. The *central tegmental tract* is an isolated bundle in the anterior part of the reticular formation containing descending pathways (mainly *rubro-olivary tracts*) and part of the very important ascending reticular formation projections to the *thalamus* and *hypothalamus*. The spinal nucleus and spinal tract of the trigeminal nerve have not changed their position, but now they are covered on the lateral side by the fibers of the middle cerebellar peduncle.

The *motor nucleus of the facial nerve* (n. VII) is immediately posterior to the superior olive and medial to the nucleus of the spinal tract of the trigeminal nerve (n. V). Before leaving the brain stem, the fibers of the facial nerve form an internal loop *(the internal genu of the facial nerve)*. The first segment of this loop courses posteromedially toward the floor of the fourth ventricle, passing close and just caudal to the *nucleus of the abducens nerve*. The facial nerve circles medially around the abducens nucleus, returning on the rostral side of the nucleus. After completing this "hairpin" bend, the nerve takes a direct course anterolaterally and slightly caudally to its exit at the pontomedullary junction. Peripherally its fibers innervate a thin sheet of branchiomeric muscles underneath the skin of the face. These are the muscles of facial expression. Fibers of the abducens nerve take a course similar to those of the hypoglossal, passing close to the lateral border of the pyramidal tract to emerge on the anterior aspect of the brain stem. These fibers innervate the lateral rectus muscle in the orbit.

The *vestibular nuclei* continue to occupy a lateral area in the floor of the fourth ventricle. The individual subnuclei at this level are the lateral, superior, and medial. The spinal (inferior) is found in the medulla.

Paired, deep cerebellar nuclei are generally observed in sections through the cerebellum at the lower level of the pons (not seen in Figure 27). These nuclei are the source of most of the neuronal outflow from the cerebellum. They include:

1. *Nucleus fastigii:* located in the midline of the roof of the fourth ventricle in the region of the vermis.
2. *Nucleus globosus:* a small group of cells located just lateral to the nucleus fastigii.
3. *Nucleus emboliformis:* a slightly elongated cellular mass located between the globose and dentate nuclei.
4. *Nucleus dentatus:* the largest and most lateral of the cerebellar nuclei. It is similar in appearance to the inferior olivary nuclear complex, purselike in shape, with an anteromedial hilum.

MIDDLE PORTION. The basilar portion of the pons is widened and thickened. The corticospinal tracts are now dispersed in separate fascicles. Mingling with them are numerous other scattered longitudinal fibers. These are the *corticopontine tracts* descending from the frontal, temporal, parietal, and occipital lobes to synapse with cells of the pontine nuclei (Fig. 28).

Two oval-shaped nuclei lie side by side in the posterolateral part of the tegmentum. The more lateral nucleus is the *main (principal) sensory nucleus of the trigeminal nerve;* the medial nucleus is the *motor nucleus of the trigeminal nerve.* Small filaments of the nerve pass posterior as the *mesencephalic root* of the trigeminal nerve. The spinal, main sensory, and mesencephalic components of the trigeminal nerve are all sensory, conveying information from pain, temperature, touch, and muscle-stretch receptors. The small motor component of V innervates the muscles of mastication. Trigeminal fibers emerging from the surface of the pons pass directly through the middle cerebellar peduncle in an anterolateral direction.

The *superior cerebellar peduncles* (brachia conjunctiva) appear at the sides of the fourth ventricle as large, compact bands (see Figs. 27 and 28). The anterior medullary velum forms the roof of the ventricle.

MIDBRAIN

The midbrain is a short segment between the pons and the diencephalon. It is traversed by the *cerebral aqueduct,* an extraordinarily small tubular passage connecting the third ventricle with the fourth.

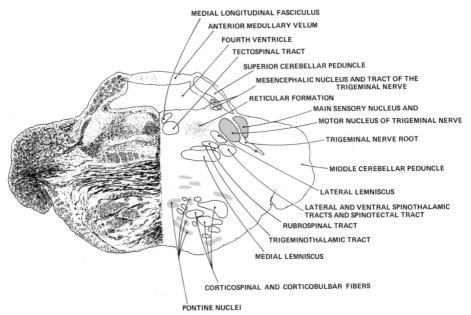

MEDIAL LONGITUDINAL FASCICULUS
ANTERIOR MEDULLARY VELUM
FOURTH VENTRICLE
TECTOSPINAL TRACT
SUPERIOR CEREBELLAR PEDUNCLE
MESENCEPHALIC NUCLEUS AND TRACT OF THE TRIGEMINAL NERVE
RETICULAR FORMATION
MAIN SENSORY NUCLEUS AND
MOTOR NUCLEUS OF TRIGEMINAL NERVE
TRIGEMINAL NERVE ROOT
MIDDLE CEREBELLAR PEDUNCLE
LATERAL LEMNISCUS
LATERAL AND VENTRAL SPINOTHALAMIC TRACTS AND SPINOTECTAL TRACT
RUBROSPINAL TRACT
TRIGEMINOTHALAMIC TRACT
MEDIAL LEMNISCUS
CORTICOSPINAL AND CORTICOBULBAR FIBERS
PONTINE NUCLEI

FIGURE 28. Cross section of the pons at the level of the main sensory and motor nuclei of V.

External Markings of the Midbrain

ANTERIOR ASPECT. The inferior surface is formed by two ropelike bundles of fibers, the *crura cerebri,* and a deep *interpeduncular fossa* that separates them (see Fig. 21). Just before it disappears within the substance of the cerebral hemisphere above, each crus cerebri is skirted by the optic tract, a continuation of fibers in the optic nerves (n. II). At its caudal end, the peduncle passes directly into the basilar portion of the pons. The oculomotor nerves (n. III) exit from the sides of the interpeduncular fossa and emerge on the surface at the transverse groove between the pons and midbrain.

POSTERIOR ASPECT. The posterior surface (tectum) of the midbrain presents four rounded elevations—the *corpora quadrigemina* (see Fig. 23). The rostral pair of swellings are the *superior colliculi,* and the somewhat smaller, caudal pair are the *inferior colliculi.* The trochlear nerves (n. IV), smallest of the cranial nerves, emerge from the posterior surface just behind the inferior colliculi after decussating in the anterior medullary velum.

Internal Structures of the Midbrain

In cross sections three zones are designated: (1) a basal portion, or crus cerebri; (2) the *tegmentum,* similar to the pontine tegmentum (the crus cerebri and the tegmentum together make up the *cerebral peduncle*); and (3) the *tectum,* or roof portion, lying above the aqueduct and forming the quadrigeminal plate.

CAUDAL HALF OF THE MIDBRAIN (LEVEL OF THE INFERIOR COLLICULUS). Each crus cerebri appears in cross section as a prominent, crescent-shaped mass of fibers within which the corticospinal and corticobulbar tracts occupy a central position, intermingled with and flanked at either side by corticopontine fibers (Fig. 29). The *substantia nigra* lies between the crus cerebri and the tegmentum. In some preparations the neurons of this area appear brown due to the melanin pigment contained within their cell bodies.

The central part of the tegmentum contains a massive interlacement of fibers—*the decussation of the superior cerebellar peduncle.* The *medial lemniscus* is displaced laterally and rotated slightly. Its outer border is in close relation to adjacent fibers of the anterolateral system. The *lateral lemniscus,* containing ascending fibers of the special sensory path of hearing, is clearly defined in the lateral part of the tegmentum posterior to the anterolateral system. Many of the fibers in the lateral lemniscus terminate dorsally in the *nucleus of the inferior colliculus.* The small, globular *nucleus of the trochlear nerve* lies near the *medial longitudinal fasciculus* in the anterior part of the central gray substance (periaqueductal gray).

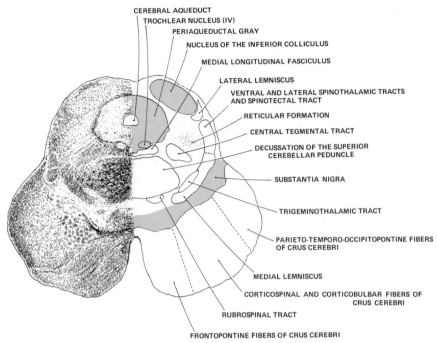

CEREBRAL AQUEDUCT
TROCHLEAR NUCLEUS (IV)
PERIAQUEDUCTAL GRAY
NUCLEUS OF THE INFERIOR COLLICULUS
MEDIAL LONGITUDINAL FASCICULUS
LATERAL LEMNISCUS
VENTRAL AND LATERAL SPINOTHALAMIC TRACTS
AND SPINOTECTAL TRACT
RETICULAR FORMATION
CENTRAL TEGMENTAL TRACT
DECUSSATION OF THE SUPERIOR
CEREBELLAR PEDUNCLE
SUBSTANTIA NIGRA
TRIGEMINOTHALAMIC TRACT
PARIETO-TEMPORO-OCCIPITOPONTINE FIBERS
OF CRUS CEREBRI
MEDIAL LEMNISCUS
CORTICOSPINAL AND CORTICOBULBAR FIBERS OF
CRUS CEREBRI
RUBROSPINAL TRACT
FRONTOPONTINE FIBERS OF CRUS CEREBRI

FIGURE 29. Cross section of the lower midbrain at the level of the inferior colliculus and decussation of the superior cerebellar peduncles.

ROSTRAL HALF OF THE MIDBRAIN (LEVEL OF THE SUPERIOR COLLICULUS). The crura cerebri and the substantia nigra continue to occupy the basal portion. The *red nuclei* are conspicuous globular masses in the anterior portion of the tegmentum (Fig. 30). The crossed fibers of the superior cerebellar peduncle pass into the red nucleus and around its edges. Many of them terminate in the red nucleus; others pass forward to the thalamus. Together these structures comprise an important part of the outflow from the cerebellum. The *tectospinal* and *rubrospinal tracts* arise from this part of the midbrain. Both tracts cross near their origin: the tectospinal in the *dorsal tegmental decussation* and the rubrospinal in the *ventral tegmental decussation*. As described earlier, both of these pathways belong to the extrapyramidal system.

The nuclear complex of the *oculomotor* nerve lies in the anterior part of the central gray matter with the *medial longitudinal fasciculus* beside it. The root fibers of the oculomotor nerve stream through and around the red nucleus before converging at their exit in the interpeduncular fossa. From there they travel to the orbit where they innervate four of the six muscles that control eye movements and one muscle that elevates the eyelid. This nerve also contains preganglionic parasympathetic fibers, which are re-

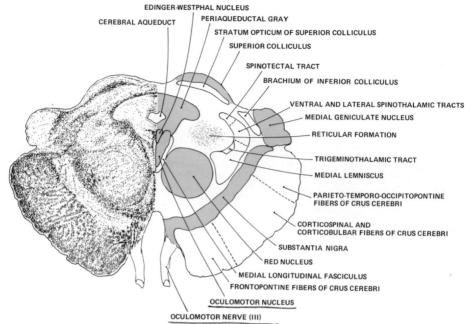

EDINGER-WESTPHAL NUCLEUS
CEREBRAL AQUEDUCT
PERIAQUEDUCTAL GRAY
STRATUM OPTICUM OF SUPERIOR COLLICULUS
SUPERIOR COLLICULUS
SPINOTECTAL TRACT
BRACHIUM OF INFERIOR COLLICULUS
VENTRAL AND LATERAL SPINOTHALAMIC TRACTS
MEDIAL GENICULATE NUCLEUS
RETICULAR FORMATION
TRIGEMINOTHALAMIC TRACT
MEDIAL LEMNISCUS
PARIETO-TEMPORO-OCCIPITOPONTINE FIBERS OF CRUS CEREBRI
CORTICOSPINAL AND CORTICOBULBAR FIBERS OF CRUS CEREBRI
SUBSTANTIA NIGRA
RED NUCLEUS
MEDIAL LONGITUDINAL FASCICULUS
FRONTOPONTINE FIBERS OF CRUS CEREBRI
OCULOMOTOR NUCLEUS
OCULOMOTOR NERVE (III)

FIGURE 30. Cross section of the upper midbrain at the level of the superior colliculus and red nucleus.

sponsible for constriction of the pupil and for changes in the shape of the lens within the eye.

The *medial geniculate bodies* appear as projections on the lateral surfaces of the midbrain. They are auditory relay centers, properly considered to be a part of the thalamus rather than the midbrain.

10

FUNCTIONAL COMPONENTS OF THE CRANIAL NERVES

The cranial nerves having functions similar to those exhibited by spinal nerves are classified as *general*. The cranial nerves having specialized functions, such as those supplying the eye and ear, conveying olfactory and gustatory impulses, or innervating the branchiomeric muscles, are classified as *special*.

SUMMARY OF FUNCTIONAL COMPONENTS

General Afferent Fibers

Sensory fibers of the general afferent type have their cells of origin in the cranial and spinal dorsal root ganglia. *General somatic afferent* (GSA) fibers carry exteroceptive (pain, temperature, and touch) and proprioceptive impulses from sensory endings in the body wall, tendons, and joints.

General visceral afferent (GVA) fibers carry sensory impulses from the visceral structures (hollow organs and glands) within the thoracic, abdominal, and pelvic cavities.

Special Afferent Fibers

Cells of origin of sensory fibers in this category are found only in the ganglia of certain cranial nerves. *Special somatic afferent* (SSA) nerves carry sensory impulses from the special sense organs in the eye and ear (vision, hearing, and equilibrium).

Special visceral afferent (SVA) fibers carry information from the olfactory and gustatory receptors. These fibers are designated as visceral because of the functional association of these sensations with the digestive tract.

General Efferent Fibers

General efferent fibers are motor fibers that arise from cells in the spinal cord and brain stem. General efferent fibers innervate all musculature of the body except the branchiomeric muscles.

General somatic efferent (GSE) fibers convey motor impulses to somatic skeletal muscles (myotomic origin). The bulk of fibers in the ventral roots of spinal nerves are of this type. In the head the somatic musculature is that of the tongue and extraocular muscles.

General visceral efferent (GVE) fibers are autonomic axons that innervate smooth and cardiac muscle fibers and regulate glandular secretion. Autonomic fibers may be subdivided into the sympathetic and parasympathetic types. Both are found in spinal nerves but parasympathetic fibers are limited. Some cranial nerves have parasympathetic components.

Special Efferent Fibers

Cranial nerves that innervate the skeletal musculature of branchiomeric origin arise from certain cranial nerve nuclei in the brain stem.

Special Visceral Efferent (SVE) fibers are nerve components that innervate striated skeletal muscles derived from the branchial arches. These muscles comprise the jaw muscles, the muscles of facial expression, and the muscles of the pharynx and larynx. The special visceral efferent fibers are not part of the autonomic nervous system.

There are no special somatic efferent fibers.

THE ANATOMIC POSITION OF CRANIAL NERVE NUCLEI IN THE BRAIN

Early in development the lateral walls of the embryonic brain and spinal cord are demarcated into an alar plate and a basal plate by the appearance of the sulcus limitans. The motor nuclei of the basal plate differentiate slightly earlier than the sensory nuclei in the alar plate. The locations of the motor and sensory cranial nerve nuclei at the level of the upper medulla are indicated and labeled according to function in Figure 31. At this level of the neuraxis the basal plate cells are medial and the alar plate cells are lateral.

Most cranial nerves contain fibers of more than one functional type, and thus most cranial nerves are associated with more than one nucleus in the brain stem. For example, the oculomotor nerve (III) contains motor fi-

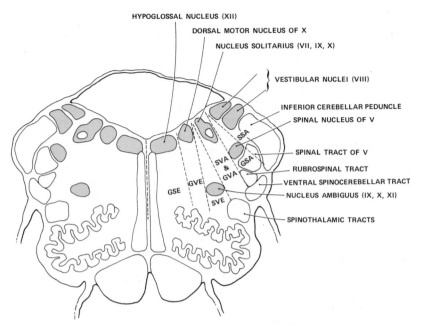

HYPOGLOSSAL NUCLEUS (XII)

DORSAL MOTOR NUCLEUS OF X

NUCLEUS SOLITARIUS (VII, IX, X)

VESTIBULAR NUCLEI (VIII)

INFERIOR CEREBELLAR PEDUNCLE

SPINAL NUCLEUS OF V

SPINAL TRACT OF V

RUBROSPINAL TRACT

VENTRAL SPINOCEREBELLAR TRACT

NUCLEUS AMBIGUUS (IX, X, XI)

SPINOTHALAMIC TRACTS

SSA

SVA & GVA

GSA

GSE

GVE

SVE

FIGURE 31. Schematic cross section of the upper medulla to show the anatomic organization of the functional cell columns *(shown in color)* that contribute motoneurons to, and receive sensory input from, the cranial nerves. Several major fiber tracts in the medulla are also labeled. GSE = general somatic efferent; GVE = general visceral efferent; SVE = special visceral efferent; SVA = special visceral afferent; GVA = general visceral afferent; GSA = general somatic afferent; SSA = special somatic afferent.

bers which originate within a general visceral efferent nucleus and a general somatic efferent nucleus in the midbrain. Its afferent fibers are associated with the mesencephalic trigeminal nucleus.

The *general somatic efferent* fibers of cranial nerves III, IV, VI, and XII arise from nuclei that are arranged as a discontinuous column of cells in the floor of the basal plate adjacent to the midline. (See the position of the nucleus of XII in Figure 31.) These nuclei are continuous with, and homologous to, the anterior horn cells of the spinal cord. They innervate musculature derived from somatic myotomes. The *general visceral efferent* nuclei of cranial nerves VII, IX, and X occupy a position lateral to the somatic efferent column. The *special visceral efferent* nuclei of cranial nerves V, VII, IX, X and XI, which provide the innervation of the branchiomeric musculature, form the most lateral discontinuous column of neurons derived from the basal lamina.

The sensory fibers of the cranial nerves arise from cell bodies in the cranial nerve ganglia. Like the central processes of cells in the dorsal root spinal ganglia, they enter the CNS and terminate in nuclei located in the alar lamina. The *visceral afferent fibers* terminate in a nuclear area adjacent to the visceral efferent column, the nucleus of the tractus solitarius. This nucleus receives *general visceral afferent* fibers in its caudal part and gustatory *(special visceral afferent)* fibers in its cephalic or rostral portion. The *general somatic afferent* column receives fibers primarily from cranial nerve V. It extends from the midbrain through the caudal extent of the medulla and into the cervical spinal cord. It consists of the mesencephalic nucleus, the principal sensory nucleus, and the nucleus of the spinal tract of V. In the spinal cord the nucleus of the spinal tract is continuous with the substantia gelatinosa. The spinal cord and cranial nerve components, which terminate in the substantia gelatinosa and the nucleus of the spinal tract of V, respectively, have the same functions—pain and temperature reception. Figure 31 indicates that the *special somatic afferent* fibers of nerve VIII terminate in the most dorsolateral portion of the alar plate of the brain stem.

Upon entering the brain stem, the functionally distinct sensory components of individual cranial nerves subdivide into fascicles that make connections with their respective, functionally distinct nuclei. For example, the central processes of the gustatory neurons of cranial nerves VII, IX, and X synapse with neurons in the cephalic portion of the solitary complex, while the somatic afferent fibers from these same nerves enter the spinal tract of V and terminate in its adjacent nucleus. Similarly, the motor nuclei of the brain stem may give rise to functional components contributing to more than one cranial nerve. The nucleus ambiguus (see Figs. 31 and 32) is the origin of the special visceral efferent fibers for IX, X, and the cranial portion of XI.

FUNCTIONAL COMPONENTS IN EACH OF THE CRANIAL NERVES

Olfactory Nerve (I)

SPECIAL VISCERAL AFFERENT. The axons of the bipolar olfactory epithelial cells constitute the olfactory nerve and terminate in the olfactory bulb.

Optic Nerve (II)

SPECIAL SOMATIC AFFERENT. The fibers (third-order neurons) that arise from the ganglion cells of the retina constitute the so-called optic nerve. It is not a true nerve but represents an evaginated fiber tract of the diencephalon. Fibers from the nasal half of each retina decussate in the optic chiasm, and beyond the chiasm these fiber bundles are called the optic tracts.

Oculomotor Nerve (III)

GENERAL SOMATIC EFFERENT. The fibers arise in the oculomotor nucleus and innervate the extrinsic muscles of the eye except for the superior oblique and lateral rectus. These muscles arise from preotic myotomes—thus the term general.

GENERAL VISCERAL EFFERENT. This functional component of III consists of the preganglionic parasympathetic fibers that arise in the accessory oculomotor (Edinger-Westphal) nucleus and terminate in the ciliary ganglion. They participate in the light and accommodation reflexes.

GENERAL SOMATIC AFFERENT. The location of the neurons of origin of proprioceptive fibers from the extrinsic ocular muscles is not entirely clear. In some species these fibers have their cell bodies of origin in the trigeminal ganglion. In others, clusters of ganglion cells have been identified along the third nerve. The central processes of these cells are thought to terminate in the trigeminal nuclear complex.

Trochlear Nerve (IV)

GENERAL SOMATIC EFFERENT. These fibers arise in the trochlear nucleus and innervate the superior oblique muscle of the eye, which is derived from the preotic myotomes.

GENERAL SOMATIC AFFERENT. The cells of origin of proprioceptive fibers from the superior oblique muscles are unknown but may be in the trigeminal ganglion.

Trigeminal Nerve (V)

GENERAL SOMATIC AFFERENT. These are of two types: exteroceptive and proprioceptive. Exteroceptive fibers from the skin of the face and scalp and the ectodermal mucous membranes of the head (mouth and nasal chamber) have their cells of origin in the trigeminal ganglion. Proprioceptive fibers from the muscles of mastication and the other muscles innervated by the mandibular nerve arise from cells in the mesencephalic nucleus of the trigeminal nerve.

SPECIAL VISCERAL EFFERENT. Fibers from the motor nucleus of the fifth nerve contribute to the mandibular nerve and innervate the muscles of mastication, tensor veli palatini, tensor tympani, mylohyoid, and the anterior belly of the digastric. These muscles arise embryologically from the first branchial arch.

Abducens Nerve (VI)

GENERAL SOMATIC EFFERENT. Fibers that arise in the abducens nucleus innervate the lateral rectus muscle of the eye, which is derived from the preotic myotomes.

GENERAL SOMATIC AFFERENT. The proprioceptive fibers from the lateral rectus muscle have unknown cells of origin, but these cells, like those contributing to the trochlear nerve, are probably located within the trigeminal ganglion and send their central processes into the trigeminal nuclear complex.

Facial Nerve (VII)

GENERAL SOMATIC AFFERENT. Cell bodies located in the geniculate ganglion have fibers conveying exteroceptive sensations (pain and temperature) from the external auditory meatus and skin of the ear. The central processes of these cells terminate in the nucleus of the spinal tract of V.

SPECIAL VISCERAL AFFERENT. Other cells in the geniculate ganglion have peripheral fibers that terminate in the taste buds on the anterior two-thirds of the tongue. The fibers reach the tongue by way of the intermediate nerve, chorda tympani, and lingual nerve. Central branches terminate in the rostral portion of the nucleus solitarius.

GENERAL VISCERAL EFFERENT. The preganglionic parasympathetic fibers, which arise in the poorly defined superior salivatory nucleus, pass through the nervus intermedius and synapse with the postganglionic neurons in the pterygopalatine and submandibular ganglia. Postganglionic fibers from these ganglia terminate in the lacrimal gland and the submandibular and sublingual salivary glands.

SPECIAL VISCERAL EFFERENT. These fibers arise from neurons in the motor nucleus of the facial nerve. They innervate the superficial muscles of the face and scalp (muscles of facial expression), platysma, stapedius, stylohyoid, and posterior belly of the digastric. These muscles originate from the second branchial arch.

Vestibulocochlear Nerve (VIII)

SPECIAL SOMATIC AFFERENT. The cochlear portion of nerve VIII has bipolar cells of origin in the spiral ganglion. Peripheral processes receive stimuli from the hair cells in the cochlear duct. The central processes terminate in the dorsal and ventral cochlear nuclei. The vestibular portion of VIII originates from bipolar neurons in the vestibular ganglion. Peripheral processes receive stimuli from hair cells in the maculae (of the utricle and saccule) and cristae (in the ampullae of the semicircular canals). The central processes terminate in four vestibular nuclei in the medulla and pons.

Glossopharyngeal Nerve (IX)

GENERAL SOMATIC AFFERENT. Cell bodies located in the superior ganglion of IX have fibers conveying exteroceptive sensations (pain and temperature) from the external auditory meatus and skin of the ear.

GENERAL VISCERAL AFFERENT. The cell bodies located in the inferior (petrosal) ganglion have peripheral fibers that carry general sensory input from the posterior third of the tongue and the pharynx. Most of the central processes terminate in the caudal part of the nucleus of the solitary tract; others probably end in the spinal nucleus of V.

SPECIAL VISCERAL AFFERENT. Other cell bodies of the inferior ganglion have peripheral fibers that carry gustatory sensations from the posterior third of the tongue. Central processes of these cells terminate in the rostral portion of the nucleus of the solitary tract.

GENERAL VISCERAL EFFERENT. Preganglionic parasympathetic fibers from cells in the inferior salivatory nucleus terminate in the otic ganglion. Postganglionic fibers of this ganglion innervate the parotid gland.

SPECIAL VISCERAL EFFERENT. Fibers originating from neurons in the nucleus ambiguus pass through branches of IX to innervate the skeletal muscle of the third visceral arch (stylopharyngeus).

Vagus nerve (X)

GENERAL SOMATIC AFFERENT. Cell bodies located in the superior (jugular) ganglion have fibers conveying exteroceptive sensations (pain and temperature) from the skin in the region of the ear. Central processes of these cells end in the spinal nucleus of V.

GENERAL VISCERAL AFFERENT. Cell bodies located in the inferior (nodose) ganglion have fibers conveying general sensations from the pharynx and larynx and from the thoracic and abdominal viscera. Central processes of these neurons terminate in the caudal part of the nucleus solitarius.

SPECIAL VISCERAL AFFERENT. Peripheral processes of other neurons in the inferior ganglion receive gustatory stimuli from epiglottal taste buds by way of the internal laryngeal nerve. These neurons also send their central processes into the nucleus solitarius, but to its more rostral regions.

GENERAL VISCERAL EFFERENT. Preganglionic parasympathetic fibers from neurons in the dorsal motor nucleus of nerve X terminate on postganglionic neurons in the visceral walls of the thoracic and abdominal viscera. Recent reports indicate that the nucleus ambiguus also gives rise to such fibers. Postganglionic fibers innervate glands, cardiac muscle, and smooth muscle.

SPECIAL VISCERAL EFFERENT. Fibers from cells in the nucleus ambiguus innervate the skeletal musculature of the remaining branchial arches (soft palate, larynx, and pharynx).

Accessory Nerve (XI)

CRANIAL PORTION

SPECIAL VISCERAL EFFERENT. Fibers arising from neurons in the nucleus ambiguus accompany those of the vagus nerve and supply the muscles of the larynx.

SPINAL PORTION

SPECIAL VISCERAL EFFERENT. Neurons in the dorsal part of the anterior horn of the upper cervical (C-2 to C-5) spinal cord give rise to fibers that exit from the cord and pass rostrally through the foramen magnum, then exit from the skull in association with cranial nerves IX and X. These fibers innervate the sternomastoid and trapezius muscles.

Hypoglossal nerve (XII)

GENERAL SOMATIC EFFERENT. Fibers from neurons in the hypoglossal nucleus innervate the skeletal musculature of the tongue, which is derived from the three occipital myotomes.

GENERAL SOMATIC AFFERENT. Proprioceptive fibers from the lingual musculature (similar to that proposed for cranial nerves III, IV, and VI) are supposed to arise from scattered neurons that have been found along the nerve.

11

CRANIAL NERVES OF THE MEDULLA

XII – Tongue → ipsi

HYPOGLOSSAL NERVE (NERVE XII)

The hypoglossal nerve is the motor nerve of the tongue. Its general somatic efferent fibers arise from lower motoneuron cell bodies in the hypoglossal nucleus. This nucleus is a column of cells extending the length of the medulla in a position just under the fourth ventricle close to the midline. Axons of these cells pass between the pyramid and the olive to exit as rootlets of the hypoglossal nerve. Among the muscles supplied by the hypoglossal nerve are the genioglossi, which draw the root of the tongue forward and cause its tip to protrude. The genioglossus muscle of each side causes the tongue, on protrusion, to deviate to the opposite side. Injury to the hypoglossal nerve on one side causes a lower motoneuron lesion with paralysis, loss of tone, and atrophy of the muscles on the side of the lesion. On voluntary protrusion, the tongue deviates to the paralyzed side.

ACCESSORY NERVE (NERVE XI)

The accessory nerve has two distinct parts. The spinal root, which arises from anterior horn cells of cervical cord segments (spinal accessory nucleus) C-2 through C-5, exits the spinal cord through the lateral funiculus as a series of rootlets, ascends through the foramen magnum, and courses along the side of the medulla. Here it joins the cranial root from the medulla. After accompanying the spinal root fibers for a short distance, the cranial fibers turn away to join the vagus nerve and are distributed with the terminal branches of the vagus to the muscles of the larynx. The spinal portion of nerve XI (special visceral efferent fibers) passes through the jugular foramen and descends in the neck to end in the sternomastoid and trapezius muscles. Injury to the spinal accessory nerve results in paralysis of the sternomastoid muscle, which causes weakness in rotating the head to the opposite side. Paralysis of the upper part of the trapezius muscle results in downward and outward rotation of the upper part of the scapula, sagging of the shoulder, and weakness in attempting to shrug the shoulder.

THE VAGAL SYSTEM (NERVES IX, X, AND PORTIONS OF NERVES VII AND XI)

Four nerves of the medulla and pons are closely related in function and in the configuration of their nuclear groups: (1) the nervus intermedius, which contains the sensory and parasympathetic fibers of the facial nerve (n. VII); (2) the glossopharyngeal nerve (n. IX); (3) the vagus nerve (n. X); and (4) the cranial portion of the accessory nerve (n. XI). These will be considered collectively as the vagal system.

The vagal system contains special visceral motor, preganglionic parasympathetic, and sensory fibers, but there is no separation of bundles into dorsal and ventral nerve roots as in the spinal nerves. All fibers enter and leave the medulla in a series of rootlets arranged in a longitudinal row posterior to the olive (Fig. 32).

We will consider three nuclear columns which contribute fibers to, or receive fibers from, these four nerves. They are (1) the special visceral motor column of the medulla, the nucleus ambiguus; (2) the preganglionic parasympathetic column, consisting of the salivatory nuclei and the dorsal motor nucleus of X; and (3) the visceral sensory column, or the nucleus of the fasciculus solitarius.

Motor Portion of the Vagal System

The cells of the *nucleus ambiguus* are lower motoneurons. Their axons enter the glossopharyngeal and vagus nerves and the cranial root of the accessory nerve to furnish motor innervation to the striated branchiomeric musculature of the soft palate, the pharynx, and the larynx (see Fig. 32).

A unilateral lesion of the vagus nerve leads to difficulty in coughing, clearing the voice, and swallowing. Frothy mucus collects in the pharynx and overflows into the larynx. The palatal arch droops on the side of the lesion. During phonation the soft palate is elevated on the normal side, and the uvula deviates to the normal side. Bilateral lesions of the vagus nerves result in difficulty swallowing (dysphagia); regurgitation of food into the nose on swallowing; difficulty producing certain vocal sounds and the development of a nasal quality to the voice (dysphonia); a tendency to mouth-

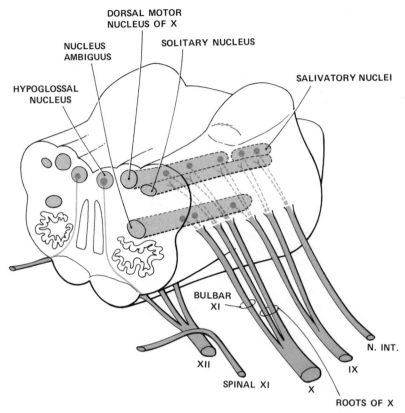

FIGURE 32. The major nuclei of the vagal system and their connections with the four nerves of that system. The hypoglossal nucleus and nerve root are also shown. N. INT. = nervus intermedius.

breathing and snoring at night; and difficulty in draining mucus from the nasal passages into the pharynx. One of the recurrent nerves carrying innervation to the larynx may be injured inadvertently during operations on the thyroid gland, resulting in transient or permanent hoarseness. Paralysis of both recurrent nerves produces stridor and dyspnea, which may necessitate tracheotomy.

Parasympathetic Portion of the Vagal System

The *dorsal motor nucleus of the vagus nerve* consists of nerve cell bodies whose axons leave the medulla and project to ganglia located in the head, neck, thorax, and abdomen. The ganglia are located close to, or within, the viscera that they innervate, and they send short fibers directly to the smooth muscle and gland cells of these organs. The fibers that arise in the dorsal motor nucleus are preganglionic parasympathetic fibers; those proceeding from the ganglia to muscle and gland cells are postganglionic.

At the rostral end of the dorsal motor nuclear column is a group of neurons belonging to the *salivatory nuclei;* activity of these cells stimulates secretion by the salivary glands. The cells in the superior salivatory nucleus send their preganglionic fibers to the nervus intermedius, while those in the inferior nucleus send preganglionic fibers to the glossopharyngeal nerve (see Fig. 32). Some of the preganglionic fibers entering the nervus intermedius terminate in the pterygopalatine ganglion. This parasympathetic ganglion sends postganglionic fibers to the lacrimal gland and to the mucosal glands of the palate, pharynx, and posterior nasal chambers. Other preganglionic fibers of the nervus intermedius end in the submandibular ganglion, which innervates the submandibular and sublingual salivary glands. Preganglionic fibers of the glossopharyngeal nerve end in the otic ganglion, the parasympathetic ganglion that innervates the parotid gland.

The dorsal motor nucleus furnishes the preganglionic fibers of the vagus nerve, the largest and most important parasympathetic nerve of the body. Ganglion cells receiving terminals of the vagus nerve are found in the autonomic plexuses of the walls of the cervical, thoracic, and abdominal viscera. Stimulation of vagal parasympathetic fibers slows the heart rate, constricts the smooth muscle of the bronchial tree, stimulates the glands of the bronchial mucosa, promotes peristalsis in the gastrointestinal tract, relaxes the pyloric and ileocolic sphincters, and stimulates the secretion of gastric and pancreatic juices.

Sensory Portion of the Vagal System

The sensory fibers of the vagus and glossopharyngeal nerves have their cell bodies in the superior and inferior sensory ganglia of each nerve. These ganglia are found near the base of the skull. The geniculate ganglion, located at the external genu of the facial nerve, contains the cell bodies of the sensory fibers of the nervus intermedius. After entering the medulla in the dorsolateral sulcus, most of the sensory fibers of the vagal system pass directly into the solitary tract. The fibers turn in a caudal direction and give off terminal branches to the nucleus of the solitary tract as they descend.

The sense of taste, initiated by chemical stimulation of special receptor cells in the taste buds of the tongue, is carried to the rostral portion of the solitary tract by sensory fibers of the nervus intermedius and the glossopharyngeal nerves. The nervus intermedius, through its chorda tympani branch, receives gustatory stimuli from the anterior two-thirds of the tongue; the glossopharyngeal, from the posterior one-third. A small number of taste buds located on the epiglottis receive innervation from the vagus nerve. Secondary fibers (the ascending gustatory tract) from the rostral portion of the nucleus of the solitary tract ascend through the brain stem on the medial aspect of the medial lemniscus to the region of the VPM nucleus of the thalamus. In most mammals these ascending solitarius fibers synapse in the parabrachial nucleus which, in turn, projects to the VPM. It is not known whether the taste pathway in the human includes this relay. Thalamic fibers go to a cortical area for taste recognition located in the opercular part of the postcentral gyrus.

The glossopharyngeal and vagus nerves supply the afferent fibers of touch and pain senses to the mucosa of the posterior part of the soft palate, middle ear cavity, auditory tube, pharynx, larynx, and trachea. These fibers, whose nerve cell bodies are in the inferior ganglia of nerves IX and X, enter the solitary tract along with the special sensory fibers of taste, but they terminate in the caudal portion of the nucleus of the solitary tract.

The vagus nerve also conducts sensory stimuli from the heart, bronchi, esophagus, stomach, small intestine, and ascending colon. Vagal stimulation may be responsible for the sensation of nausea, but otherwise, afferent impulses from viscera are not recognized consciously when they are conducted by the vagal route. Visceral pain is transmitted by the anterolateral system of the spinal cord, which receives its input from visceral afferents accompanying the sympathetic nerves. The chief function of the nontaste, afferent fibers of the vagal system concerns the operation of visceral reflexes.

Somatic sensation (pain, touch, temperature) from the skin of the posterior part of the auricle is transmitted to the brain stem over fibers whose cell bodies are in the superior ganglia of IX and X and the geniculate ganglion of VII. Upon entering the brain stem, the central processes of these cells are believed to enter the spinal tract of V and to terminate, along with the other fibers in that tract, on cells in the adjacent nucleus of the spinal tract. This functional component of the vagal system is not illustrated in Figure 32.

Course and Distribution of Nerves of the Vagal System

NERVUS INTERMEDIUS

The nervus intermedius, the smaller of two divisions of the facial nerve, exits from the brain stem at the junction of the medulla and pons. It enters the internal acoustic meatus and proceeds laterally in the facial canal toward the medial wall of the middle ear cavity. The sensory ganglion (geniculate ganglion) is located at the angle of a sharp bend in the canal. From this point, some fibers of the nerve continue as the greater superficial petrosal nerve to the pterygopalatine ganglion. The rest of the nervus intermedius passes downward in the facial canal but leaves it abruptly and crosses the tympanic cavity as the chorda tympani. Leaving the middle ear at the medial end of the petrotympanic fissure, the chorda tympani descends between the pterygoid muscles to join the lingual branch of the mandibular division of the trigeminal nerve. Some fibers of the chorda tympani are given off to the submandibular ganglion, and the rest are distributed to taste receptors in the anterior two-thirds of the tongue.

GLOSSOPHARYNGEAL NERVE

The glossopharyngeal nerve leaves the skull through the jugular foramen where its two sensory ganglia, superior and inferior, are located. The nerve passes downward and forward to be distributed to the stylopharyngeus muscle and the mucosa of the palatine tonsil, the fauces, and to the posterior one-third of the tongue.

The glossopharyngeal nerve has five branches:

1. The *tympanic* branch enters the tympanic plexus, provides innervation to the membranes of the tympanic cavity, proceeds from the plexus as the lesser superficial petrosal nerve, and terminates in the otic ganglion.
2. The *carotid* branch descends along the internal carotid artery to the carotid sinus and the carotid body.
3. The *pharyngeal* branch enters the pharyngeal plexus with the vagus nerve and supplies the mucous membrane of the pharynx with sensory branches.
4. The *stylopharyngeal* branch consists of motor fibers to the stylopharyngeus muscle.
5. The *lingual* branch sends taste and general sensory fibers to the posterior third of the tongue.

VAGUS NERVE

The two sensory ganglia of the vagus nerve, the superior (jugular) and inferior (nodose), are located near the jugular foramen through which the nerve passes. The nerve courses down the neck in the carotid sheath and enters the thorax, passing anterior to the subclavian artery on the right and anterior to the aortic arch on the left. Both nerves pass behind the roots of the lungs. The left nerve continues on the anterior side and the right nerve on the posterior side of the esophagus to reach the gastric plexus. Fibers diverge from this plexus to the duodenum, liver, biliary ducts, spleen, kidneys, and to the small and large intestine as far as the splenic flexure.

The vagus nerve has several branches:

1. The *auricular* branch extends to skin in the external auditory canal and a small sector of the pinna. (The central connections of this branch may be to the nucleus of the spinal tract of V.)
2. The *pharyngeal* branch extends to the pharyngeal plexus, along with the glossopharyngeal nerve. It is the chief motor nerve of the pharynx and soft palate.

3. The *superior laryngeal* internal branch is sensory to mucosa of the larynx and epiglottis; its external branch innervates inferior pharyngeal constrictor and cricothyroid muscles.
4. The *recurrent laryngeal* branch, on the left side, loops around the aortic arch from before backwards; on the right side, it takes a similar course around the subclavian artery. Both nerves ascend in the laryngotracheal grooves and supply motor fibers to the intrinsic muscles of the larynx and sensory fibers to the mucosa below the vocal cords.
5. The *cardiac* (superior and inferior cervical cardiac rami and thoracic) branches enter the cardiac plexus on the wall of the heart with cardiac nerves from the sympathetic trunks.
6. The *pericardial, bronchial, esophageal,* and other branches divide to enter the pulmonary, celiac, superior mesenteric, and other plexi to the thoracic and abdominal viscera.

CRANIAL ACCESSORY NERVE

The cranial accessory nerve joins the vagus nerve and contributes to the laryngeal branches of that nerve.

Reflexes of the Vagal System

SALIVARY-TASTE REFLEX

The secretory function of the vagal system is illustrated by the salivary-taste reflex. When a gustatory stimulus such as a drop of weak acid is placed on the anterior two-thirds of the tongue, the salivary glands increase their output of saliva. The afferent stimulus is carried by the facial nerve to the nucleus of the solitary tract by taste fibers. Connecting fibers from this nucleus go to parasympathetic neurons in the superior and inferior salivatory nuclei, which supply the salivary glands through the facial and glossopharyngeal nerves.

CAROTID SINUS REFLEX

Increased blood pressure stimulates special baroreceptors in the wall of the carotid sinus and sends impulses over afferent fibers of the glossopharyngeal nerve to the solitary tract. Connections from the solitary tract, through a synapse in its nucleus, to the dorsal motor nucleus and efferent fibers of the vagus nerve complete a reflex arc that slows the heart rate. Simultaneously, other reflex connections are made to a diffuse vasomotor "center" located in the reticular formation of the medulla. Inhibition of the vasomotor center, whose fibers descend to sympathetic neurons of the spinal cord, produces vasodilation of peripheral blood vessels and further reduces the blood pressure. Some individuals with hypersensitive carotid sinus reflexes are subject to attacks of syncope brought on by light external pressure over the sinus.

CAROTID BODY REFLEX

The carotid body contains special chemoreceptors that respond to changes in the carbon dioxide and oxygen content of the circulating blood. Activation of these chemoreceptors sends impulses through the glosso-pharyngeal nerve to the solitary tract. Fibers then go to the respiratory center of the medulla where they influence the rate of respiration. The respiratory center consists of diffusely arranged cells of the reticular forma-tion with reticulospinal fibers descending to the lower motoneurons of the phrenic and intercostal nerves.

Propagation of nerve impulses over the reticulospinal fibers from the respiratory center produces inspiration. As the lungs become inflated, stretch receptors in the walls of bronchioles discharge impulses that as-cend to the medulla through the vagus nerve. Connecting neurons reach the respiratory center and, by inhibition, temporarily arrest the inspiratory phase of respiration. The respiratory center depends on impulses descend-ing from the pons for maintenance of the rhythm. The activity of neurons in the respiratory center can be controlled voluntarily for acts such as singing and talking.

COUGH REFLEX

Coughing is usually a response to irritation of the larynx, trachea, or bron-chial tree, but it may also be produced at times by stimulation of vagus nerve fibers in other locations, including the external auditory canal or the tympanic membrane. Afferent impulses reach the solitary nucleus and tract by way of the vagus nerve. Connections are made to the respiratory center to bring about forced expiration. At the same time, fibers going to the nu-cleus ambiguus cause efferent impulses to descend to the muscles of the larynx and pharynx for their participation in coughing.

GAG REFLEX

Touching the posterior wall of the pharynx results in constriction and eleva-tion of the pharynx. The afferent fibers for this reflex are sensory fibers of the glossopharyngeal nerve. After entering the solitary tract they make syn-aptic connections with the nucleus ambiguus, which sends efferent fibers to the striated muscles of the pharynx.

VOMITING REFLEX

Forceful emptying of the stomach is brought about by relaxation of the gastroesophageal sphincter and contraction of the muscles of the anterior abdominal wall, which expel gastric contents. At the same time, inspiration is arrested by closure of the glottis. The stimulus, which may arise in any part of the gut innervated by the vagus nerve, evokes impulses sent to the nucleus of the solitary tract by sensory fibers of the vagus nerve. From here impulses go to the dorsal motor nucleus to initiate the parasympathetic responses, to the nucleus ambiguus to close the glottis, and to neurons of the medullary reticular formation. Impulses in the reticular formation descend into the spinal cord and activate the appropriate lower motoneurons to cause contraction of the diaphragm and abdominal muscles.

A general elevation of intracranial pressure can cause vomiting. This probably results from transmission of the increased pressure onto the floor of the fourth ventricle. Vomiting can occur also if there is localized pressure on the medulla from a pathologic process such as a local tumor or hemorrhage.

12

CRANIAL NERVES OF THE PONS AND MIDBRAIN

ABDUCENS NERVE (NERVE VI)

The abducens nerve, arising from its nucleus beneath the fourth ventricle in the pons, supplies the motor fibers of the *lateral rectus muscle* of the eye. Leaving the brain stem anteriorly at the junction of the medulla and pons, the nerve passes along the floor of the posterior fossa of the skull to reach the lateral wall of the cavernous sinus. The nerve can be damaged in the brain stem or in its long intracranial course. In addition, prolonged elevation of intracranial pressure from any cause may damage the abducens nerve. Sustaining such damage makes it impossible to turn the eye outward. The unopposed pull of the medial rectus muscle causes the eye to turn inward (adduct), thereby producing *internal strabismus,* or squint. In cases in which only one of the two nerves is involved, images do not fall on corresponding points of the left and right retinae; as a result, they cannot be fused properly. The result is diplopia, or double vision, which worsens when the patient attempts to gaze to the side of the lesion. The two images are seen side by side, and thus the disorder is termed *horizontal diplopia.* The patient usually attempts to minimize the diplopia by rotating the head so that the chin turns toward the side of the lesion. With bilateral abducens nerve paralysis, both eyes are turned inward and neither eye can be moved in a lateral direction past the midposition.

TROCHLEAR NERVE (NERVE IV)

The nucleus of the trochlear nerve is located anterior to the central gray matter in the region of the inferior colliculus. The fibers of the nerve descend slightly and curve around the central gray matter. The fibers decussate in the anterior medullary velum and make their exit from the posterior surface of the tectum caudal to the inferior colliculus. The trochlear nerve innervates the superior oblique muscle. The muscle has its strongest action when its tendon of insertion is parallel to the sagittal axis of the globe. Thus an isolated lesion of the trochlear nerve results in loss of downward ocular movement when the eye is turned toward the nose. The patient with an isolated trochlear nerve lesion complains of vertical diplopia and tilts his head in order to align the eyes and thereby eliminate the diplopia.

OCULOMOTOR NERVE (NERVE III)

The nucleus of the oculomotor nerve is located anterior to the central gray matter in the region of the superior colliculus. The fibers course ventrally, some penetrating the lateral portion of the red nucleus and the medial portion of the cerebral peduncle. After its exit from the brain stem at the interpeduncular fossa, the nerve passes close to the arteries of the circle of Willis, which is an anastomotic circuit at the base of the brain. An aneurysm (saccular dilation) in one of the arteries in this region may compress the oculomotor nerve. Tumor or hemorrhage may push the inferior margin of the temporal lobe under the edge of the tentorium cerebelli and exert pressure on the oculomotor nerve as it crosses the tentorium.

The oculomotor nerve innervates the *medial, superior* and *inferior recti,* the *inferior oblique,* and the *levator palpebrae superioris.* Each of these muscles is innervated by fibers from its own subgroup of neurons in the oculomotor nuclear complex. The three recti and the inferior oblique receive input only from neurons on the same side of the brain stem, but each levator palpebrae is innervated by axons of cells in both the right and left nuclei. A special subgroup of cells in this complex, the Edinger-Westphal nucleus, contributes *preganglionic parasympathetic fibers to the ciliary ganglion* whose postganglionic fibers innervate the *ciliary muscle for accommodation* and the *sphincter muscle of the iris,* which constricts the pupil.

Lesions of the oculomotor nerve cause an ipsilateral lower motoneuron paralysis of the muscles supplied by the nerve. This results in (1) outward deviation (abduction) of the eye *(external strabismus)* and inability to turn the eye vertically or inward; (2) *ptosis,* or drooping of the upper eyelid, with inability to raise the lid voluntarily; and (3) dilation of the pupil *(mydriasis)* because of the unopposed action of the radial muscle fibers of the iris, which are supplied by the sympathetic system. Incomplete lesions produce partial effects. There may be some weakness of all functions, or one symptom may appear without the others (e.g., dilation of the pupil without paralysis of eye movements). Patients with diabetes mellitus are prone to develop vascular lesions of the oculomotor nerve with loss of all functions except for pupillary responses.

The upper motoneurons which descend from the cerebral cortex to the motor nuclei of nerves III, IV, and VI originate in area 8 of the frontal lobe and project to the superior colliculus ipsilaterally. Second-order neurons project to the opposite side of the nervous system in the pons and, through the paramedian pontine reticular formation, make connections with all three nuclei to bring about cooperative, or conjugate, movements of both eyes. Upper motoneuron lesions, therefore, usually do not affect one nerve without involving the others. The cortex of the left frontal lobe controls voluntary deviation of the eyes to the right. Destructive lesions above the crossing of the corticobulbar tract cause loss of the ability to turn the eyes voluntarily to the side opposite the lesion. Following such a lesion, the predominating influence of the unaffected corticobulbar tracts may cause both eyes to be deviated to the side of the lesion so that the patient "looks at his lesion."

frontal eye fields

FACIAL NERVE (NERVE VII)

The motor division of the seventh cranial nerve is considered to be the facial nerve proper, since its sensory and parasympathetic components (nervus intermedius) are included with the vagal system. The facial is the motor nerve of the muscles of facial expression *(mimetic muscles)*. Through the action of the orbicularis oculi muscle, the facial nerve closes the eyelid and protects the eye.

The facial nerve arises from nerve cell bodies in the facial nucleus of the pontine tegmentum (see Figs. 27 and 33). The neuronal cell groups in this nucleus are subdivided according to the particular muscles that they innervate. The fibers emerging from these neurons proceed from the cerebellopontine angle, enter the facial canal, leave the skull by the stylomastoid foramen, and course through the substance of the parotid gland behind the ramus of the mandible where they divide into branches that fan out to the face and scalp.

Loss of function of the facial nerve causes total paralysis of the muscles of facial expression on that side. The muscles of one side of the face sag, and the normal lines around the lips, nose, and forehead are "ironed out." When the patient attempts to smile, the corner of the mouth is drawn to the opposite side, and saliva may ooze from the lips on the paralyzed side. The cheek may puff out in expiration because the buccinator muscle is paralyzed. Although corneal sensation persists, the corneal reflex is lost on the side of the lesion because the motor fibers involved in this reflex do not function. The patient's inability to close his eyes on the side of the paralysis leads to irritation of the cornea and predisposes to infection; thus he needs to use protective eye drops and wear a bandage over the eye. It is not uncommon for the facial nerve to lose function overnight without any known cause except for marked swelling with compression of the nerve in the bony facial canal, a condition known as Bell's palsy. Fortunately, most patients with Bell's palsy recover spontaneously in one or two months.

Because there are no stretch reflexes available for testing the superficial musculature of the face, these cannot be used to distinguish an upper motoneuron lesion from a lower motoneuron lesion causing weakness of the facial muscles. An upper motoneuron lesion usually can be recognized by other means. Nearly all of the axons projecting from the cerebral cortex to the neurons of the facial nucleus that supply the lower part of the face (below the angle of the eye) are crossed fibers; uncrossed as well as crossed fibers project to motor cells for the upper part of the face (Fig. 33). In consequence, an upper motoneuron lesion interrupts the voluntary control fibers for lower facial muscles but leaves an uncrossed connection open for movements of the upper facial muscles. As a result, the upper part of the face is spared from paralysis.

When paralysis results from injury to upper motoneurons rather than to the facial nerve itself or its nucleus, involuntary contraction of the muscles of facial expression remains possible. In response to an emotional stimulus, the muscles of the lower face will contract symmetrically when the patient smiles or laughs. This is because the neural mechanism for emotional facial expression is separate from that for voluntary facial movement. The anatomic pathways mediating emotional facial expression are unknown.

TRIGEMINAL NERVE (NERVE V)

The trigeminal nerve is a mixed nerve with a large motor root supplying the muscles of mastication and an even larger sensory root distributed to the face, mouth, nasal cavity, orbit, and anterior half of the scalp.

Motor Division of Nerve V

Fibers from the masticator, or motor nucleus, in the lateral tegmentum of the rostral pons enter the mandibular branch of the fifth nerve and innervate the temporalis, masseter, and medial and lateral pterygoid muscles (other smaller muscles are also supplied). Peripheral lesions of this portion of the nerve cause atrophy and weakness, which can be recognized by feeling the size and tautness of the masseter muscles as the jaws are clenched. Fasciculations may be seen in the denervated muscle fibers. Owing to the action of the pterygoid muscles that draw the mandible forward and toward the midline, the chin deviates in the direction of the paralyzed side when the jaw opens. The motor nucleus of each side receives input from upper motoneurons originating in both the left and the right motor areas of the cortex, and supranuclear lesions confined to one side do not produce any marked effects. The jaw jerk is a stretch reflex obtained by placing the examiner's index finger over the middle of the patient's chin with the patient's mouth slightly open and tapping the finger gently with a

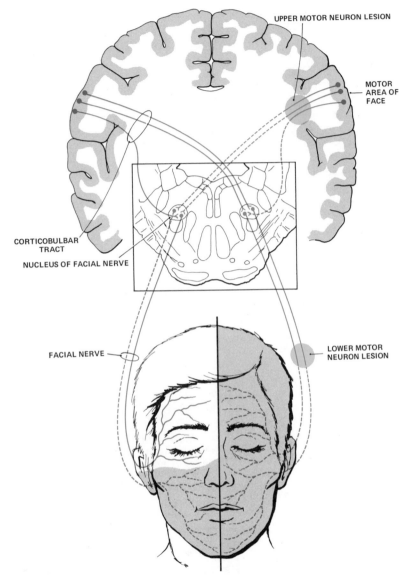

FIGURE 33. The shaded areas of the face show the distribution of the facial muscles paralyzed after a supranuclear lesion of the corticobulbar tract (upper motoneuron lesion) and after a lesion of the facial nerve (lower motoneuron lesion).

reflex hammer. The normal response is a slight contraction of the masseter and temporalis muscles bilaterally, causing the jaw to close slightly. This response can become exaggerated by upper motoneuron lesions rostral to the level of the pons.

Sensory Division of Nerve V

The *trigeminal* (semilunar, gasserian) *ganglion* contains cell bodies of the afferent fibers of the fifth nerve with the exception of the proprioceptive fibers from neuromuscular spindles. The proprioceptive fibers project to the *mesencephalic nucleus,* which is located in the dorsolateral part of the tegmentum of the pons and the lateral periaqueductal gray of the midbrain (Fig. 34). Unipolar nerve cell bodies of the proprioceptive fibers of the trigeminal nerve are unique in that they are located within the central nervous system. Fibers mediating the sensations of pain and temperature turn caudally after entering the pons and form the *spinal tract of the trigeminal nerve,* giving off terminal branches to the *nucleus of the spinal tract of V* as they descend through the pons and medulla. Fibers arising from cells of the nucleus of the spinal tract cross to the opposite side of the brain stem as the *ventral trigeminothalamic tract* and ascend to the medial part of the *ventral posteromedial (VPM) nucleus* of the thalamus from which thalamocortical fibers project to the postcentral gyrus. In the medulla, the crossed pain and temperature fibers of the face are located near the medial lemniscus; as they reach the pons, they gradually shift laterally to join the lateral spinothalamic tract. Fibers mediating tactile sensation project to the principal sensory nucleus (see Fig. 34) and the rostral part of the nucleus of the spinal tract. These nuclei give off both crossed and uncrossed fibers that form the *dorsal trigeminothalamic tract.* The name *trigeminal lemniscus* is sometimes applied to all of the trigeminothalamic fibers, although they are never gathered into a distinct and separate bundle.

Lesions in the lateral part of the medulla or lower pons that damage the spinal tract of the trigeminal nerve are likely to include the lateral spinothalamic tract as well. This causes loss of pain and temperature sense on the same side of the face as the lesion, and loss of pain and temperature sense on the opposite side of the body beginning at the neck. In the upper pons and midbrain, the fibers mediating pain, temperature, touch, joint position sense, and vibration sense are all close together, and in these regions one lesion produces anesthesia of the opposite side of the body including the face.

When the cornea is touched by a foreign body such as a wisp of cotton, the *corneal reflex* produces prompt closing of the eyelids. Sensory fibers entering the upper part of the spinal tract of V synapse with cells of the nucleus of the spinal tract, which send axons to the nucleus of the facial nerve. Motor fibers of the facial nerve then activate the orbicularis oculi muscle to close the eye on the side that had been touched. Connecting fibers from the nucleus of the spinal tract go to the facial nucleus of the

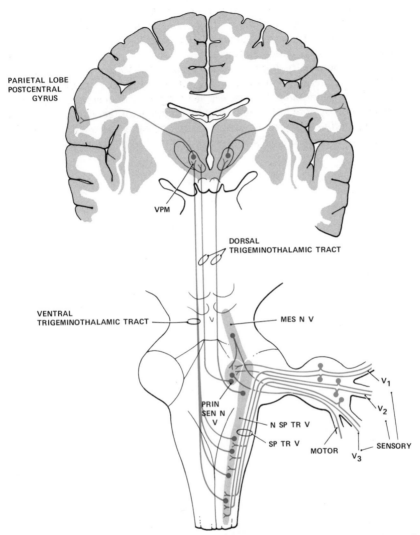

FIGURE 34. Schematic dorsal view of the brain stem showing the connections of the afferent and efferent fibers of the trigeminal nerve. V-1 = ophthalmic nerve; V-2 = maxillary nerve; V-3 = mandibular nerve; MES NV = mesencephalic nucleus of V; PRIN SEN N V = principal sensory nucleus of V; N SP TR V = nucleus of the spinal tract of V; SP TR V = spinal tract of V; VPM = ventral posteromedial nucleus of the thalamus.

opposite side to close the eye on that side as well. The response on the side that is stimulated is the *direct corneal reflex;* that in the other eye is the *consensual corneal reflex.* Interrupting the trigeminal nerve abolishes both responses. A consensual reflex will be obtained if the ipsilateral facial nerve is destroyed, but at the same time, reflex connections are made with autonomic neurons to produce increased lacrimation.

Tic douloureux, or *trigeminal neuralgia,* is a disorder characterized by attacks of unbearably severe pain over the distribution of one or more branches of the trigeminal nerve. A small trigger zone may be present, and its stimulation by light touch, temperature changes, or facial movement may set off a painful paroxysm. No cause for the disease has been discovered, but medical therapy can relieve the symptoms in most patients.

13

HEARING

THE AUDITORY SYSTEM

The eighth cranial nerve is the original sensory nerve of the semicircular canals of fish—an effective mechanism for maintaining equilibrium and orientation in space.

The essential auditory organ, initially the lagena and then the cochlea, developed gradually in the labyrinth of land vertebrates. Because of this evolutionary change, a new exteroceptive division of the eighth nerve appeared in order to serve auditory functions. Thus the eighth nerve has two components: a vestibular and a cochlear division. Both are so distinct in their function and anatomic relationships that they could be considered as separate cranial nerves.

The auditory apparatus consists of three components: the external, middle, and internal ear. There are three spaces in the skull that are separated from one another solely by membranes (see Fig. 35A). The external ear, or *external auditory meatus,* is separated from the cavity of the middle ear by the *tympanic membrane,* which receives airborne vibrations. A chain of three ossicles (malleus, incus, and stapes) spans the middle ear (see Fig. 35B). The first, the *malleus,* is attached to the tympanic membrane. The last, the *stapes,* has a footplate that fits into the oval window between the middle and inner ear cavities. The stapes is secured to the margin of the oval window by a ligament that seals this window and separates the air-filled middle ear from the fluid-filled inner ear.

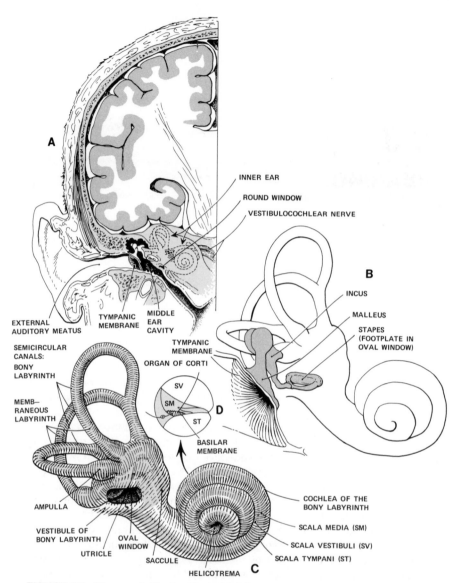

FIGURE 35. The ear. *A.* The location of the three parts of the ear (external, middle, and inner) in relation to the skull and the brain. *B.* The relationship of the ear drum (tympanic membrane) and three bones (ossicles) in the middle ear that connect it to the inner ear. *C.* The bony labyrinth, and the membranous labyrinth *(color)* within it, forming the inner ear. *D.* A cross section through the bony and membranous labyrinths of the cochlea to show the location of the organ of Corti within the membranous labyrinth.

The chain of three ossicles in the middle ear serves as an amplifier as well as an impedance-matching device that decreases the amount of energy lost by the sound waves (compressions and rarefactions) in going from the air to the fluid *(perilymph)* behind the oval window. The oval window is an opening into the *vestibule* portion of the inner ear (see Fig. 35C). Continuous with the perilymph-filled vestibule is the *cochlea,* a tube resembling a snail shell, about 3.5 cm long, and exhibiting 2½ turns. The vestibule and cochlea constitute two of the three chambers of the inner ear. The third is the set of *semicircular canals,* which will be discussed further in the next chapter. These three connected chambers within the temporal bone of the skull make up the *bony labyrinth.* Within this perilymph-filled bony cavity lies a *membranous labyrinth,* which is similar in shape to the bony labyrinth (except in the vestibule), and which is filled with another fluid—the *endolymph.*

In the cochlear part of the bony labyrinth, the central bony core or *modiolus* provides support for the bony spiral lamina, which partially divides the cochlea into two perilymphatic chambers: the *scala vestibuli* and the *scala tympani.* The membranous labyrinth within the cochlea is called the *scala media,* or cochlear duct. Stretching across the cochlea from the spiral lamina to the opposite wall of the cochlea, this cochlear duct completes the separation of the scala vestibuli and scala tympani. The *organ of Corti,* which contains the sensory epithelium or hair cells, stretches along the length of the cochlear duct, resting on the basilar membrane as it spirals around the turns of the cochlea.

The piston action of the stapes produces an instantaneous pressure wave in the perilymph of the *scala vestibuli* that travels to the *helicotrema* (the apical connection between the scala vestibuli and tympani) in 25 microseconds. A traveling wave is set up on the basilar membrane as a result of the pressure wave in the perilymph of the scala vestibuli. The basilar membrane is narrower at the base of the cochlea (near the vestibule) than at the apex; thus the mechanical properties of the basilar membrane, upon which the organ of Corti is located, vary gradually from base to apex. As a result, the pressure wave produced by a sound of a specific frequency (pitch) causes the basilar membrane to vibrate maximally at a particular point along its length. Shearing forces on the hairs of the hair cells created by this vibration lead to ionic fluxes in the closely applied dendritic processes of the spiral ganglion cells. The *spiral ganglion,* located in the modiolus of the cochlea, contains the bipolar cells of the cochlear division of the eighth nerve.

The organ of Corti serves as an audiofrequency analyzer. It is tonotopically organized so that the highest tones (highest in pitch and frequency) maximally stimulate the hair cells in the most basal portion of the cochlea, where the basilar membrane is narrow. The tones of lowest pitch maximally stimulate the most apical hair cells. Tones or sounds of intermediate pitch stimulate the hair cells in the intermediate portion of the basilar membrane. The pressure waves, after traversing through the scala media, across the basilar membrane, and through the scala tympani, are damped at the *round window.*

THE AUDITORY PATHWAY

The cochlear nerve enters the brain stem at the junction of the medulla and pons. As it attaches to the brain stem, the nerve clings to the lateral side of the inferior cerebellar peduncle and enters the *posterior (dorsal) and anterior (ventral) cochlear nuclei.* The entering nerve fibers bifurcate and make synapses with both cochlear nuclei. The nuclei are tonotopically organized. Three projections, the acoustic striae, arise from the cochlear nuclei to relay the information centrally and rostrally. The *dorsal acoustic stria* originates in the posterior cochlear nucleus, passes over the inferior cerebellar peduncle, and crosses to join the contralateral *lateral lemniscus* (Fig. 36). The two other striae arise from the anterior cochlear nucleus. The *intermediate acoustic stria* takes a course which is similar to that of the dorsal stria. The *ventral acoustic stria* takes a different route and passes anterior to the inferior cerebellar peduncle to terminate in the ipsilateral and contralateral *nuclei of the trapezoid body* and *superior olivary nuclei.* These nuclei project fibers into the ipsilateral and contralateral lateral lemnisci. Fibers in the lateral lemniscus ascend through the brain stem to terminate in the *nucleus of the inferior colliculus* and the medial geniculate nucleus. Some of the fibers terminate in small nuclear groups, the *nuclei of the lateral lemniscus,* which are intermingled with the lateral lemniscus. Some fibers of the lateral lemniscus pass directly to the medial geniculate body as the central acoustic tract, while others terminate in the *nucleus of the inferior colliculus,* which sends axons to the *medial geniculate* body through the *brachium of the inferior colliculus.*

The medial geniculate bodies are the final sensory relay stations of the hearing path, special sensory nuclei of the thalamus. The efferent connection of the medial geniculate body to the temporal lobe forms the auditory radiation which goes to the *anterior transverse temporal gyrus (gyrus of Heschl)* located on the dorsal surface of the superior temporal convolution and partly buried in the lateral fissure. This relatively small cortical region, area 41, is the primary auditory receptive area. When auditory impulses arrive at area 41, a sound is heard, but mammals, including man, can make discriminations of differing frequencies and intensities without an intact auditory cortex. This area appears to be essential, however, for discriminations requiring a response to changes in the temporal patterning of sounds, and for recognition of the location or direction of a sound. The processing of information about the location of a sound may occur primarily in the part of the pathway including the superior olive, inferior colliculus, and auditory cortex, while evaluation of meaningful combinations of different frequencies in a temporal sequence may occur in the cochlear nuclei, medial geniculate nucleus, and auditory cortex. A tonotopic organization has been demonstrated for all of these central auditory nuclei, but as indicated

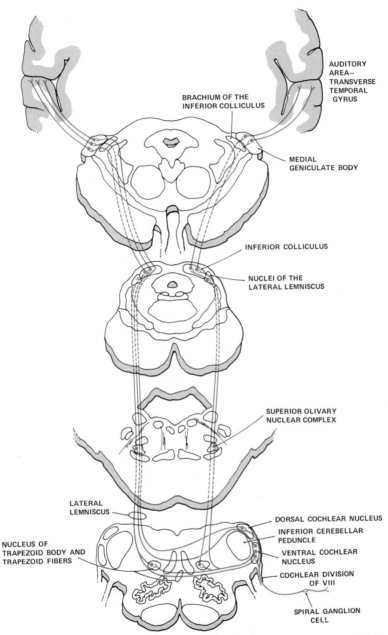

AUDITORY
AREA—
TRANSVERSE
TEMPORAL
GYRUS

BRACHIUM OF THE
INFERIOR COLLICULUS

MEDIAL
GENICULATE BODY

INFERIOR COLLICULUS

NUCLEI OF THE
LATERAL LEMNISCUS

SUPERIOR OLIVARY
NUCLEAR COMPLEX

LATERAL
LEMNISCUS

DORSAL COCHLEAR NUCLEUS

INFERIOR CEREBELLAR
PEDUNCLE

NUCLEUS OF
TRAPEZOID BODY AND
TRAPEZOID FIBERS

VENTRAL COCHLEAR
NUCLEUS

COCHLEAR DIVISION
OF VIII

SPIRAL GANGLION
CELL

FIGURE 36. The auditory pathways. Axons of neurons in the cochlear nuclei actually cross the midline as they ascend, so that they enter the lateral lemniscus at the level of the pontomedullary junction. Here they are shown crossing completely in the medulla, for diagrammatic convenience.

above, this information may be used for analysis of a variety of significant properties of sound in addition to recognition of tones.

Descending efferent fibers have been found in all parts of the auditory pathway. It is believed that they function as feedback loops. An olivocochlear bundle (from the superior olive to the ipsilateral and contralateral organ of Corti by the eighth nerve) may have an inhibitory action on the impulses from the cochlea, or may play a role in controlling metabolic processes in the cochlear duct that affect the function of the hair cells.

Bilateral Representation of the Ears in Each Temporal Lobe

Above the level at which the cochlear nerve enters the brain stem, the hearing pathway is made up of crossed and uncrossed fibers, the majority of which are crossed. Opportunity for auditory information to be redistributed in both crossed and uncrossed fashion exists at many levels of the brain stem. Fibers crossing from one side to the other occur between the superior olivary nuclei, the nuclei of the trapezoid body, the nuclei of the lateral lemnisci, and the nuclei of the inferior colliculi. These commissural connections are not illustrated in Figure 36. Each lateral lemniscus, therefore, conducts stimuli from both ears. A lesion of the right lateral lemniscus, or of the right anterior transverse temporal gyrus, stops some impulses from both ears but does not interfere with other impulses from both ears going to the cortex of the left hemisphere. Deafness in one ear usually signifies trouble in the acoustic nerve, the cochlea, or the sound-conducting apparatus of the middle ear on that side. The eighth nerve can be damaged bilaterally by toxic effects of some drugs, the most notorious being streptomycin, quinine, and aspirin.

HEARING DEFECTS FROM NERVE DAMAGE AND FROM CONDUCTION DEFECTS

Injury to fibers of the eighth nerve commonly produces hearing loss and tinnitus (ringing or roaring in the ear). These disturbances may be caused also by lesions involving the auditory conducting mechanisms in the middle ear, a condition termed conduction deafness.

Examination with a tuning fork is helpful in distinguishing nerve deafness from conduction deafness. A 256-cycle-per-second tuning fork should be used. In *Weber's test,* the base of the vibrating tuning fork is applied to the forehead in the midline, and the patient is asked whether the sound is heard in the midline or is localized in one ear. In normal individuals the sound appears to be in the midline. In a patient with conduction deafness the sound seems louder in the affected ear, and in nerve deafness it seems louder in the normal ear. This is because, in nerve deafness, bone conduction of sound is as ineffective in stimulating the damaged nerve as is air conduction. By contrast, in conduction deafness, air conduction is reduced but bone conduction is relatively enhanced.

Rinne's test compares the patient's ability to hear a vibrating tuning fork by bone conduction and by air conduction. The base of the vibrating tuning fork is placed over the mastoid process of the skull. When it can be heard no longer, it is removed and the tines are held in front of the ear. A normal person continues to hear by air conduction after bone conduction ceases. In nerve deafness, both are diminished, but air conduction remains better than bone conduction. In conduction deafness, bone conduction is better than air conduction.

Audiometers provide refined testing of hearing since pure tones may be used at controlled intensities. Receivers for both air and bone conduction are available, and it is possible to graph the results of these tests in each ear for both air and bone conduction. Conduction deafness generally is indicated by an impairment in reception of the lower frequencies of pure tones in the air conduction test. In nerve deafness tested in the same manner, the threshold deficit occurs in the reception of tones in the higher frequencies.

Nerve deafness commonly occurs with Menière's disease, trauma, damage by drugs, infection, aging, and occlusion of the internal auditory artery. Conduction deafness may result from wax in the external auditory canal, otitis media, and diseases that impair the capacity of the ossicles to function properly.

AUDITORY REFLEXES

Auditory reflexes are operated by side branches from the main auditory pathway. Many of these synapse in the reticular formation to evoke autonomic responses. Fibers from the inferior colliculus to the superior colliculus provide auditory input to the spinal cord as components of the *tectospinal tract*. These fibers terminate on lower motoneurons in the cervical spinal cord supplying the muscles of the head and neck that respond to sound.

14

THE VESTIBULAR SYSTEM

The vestibular part of the eighth nerve has its peripheral endings on the hair cells of both the maculae of the utricle and saccule, and on the cristae in the ampullae of the three semicircular canals (see Fig. 35). The nerve furnishes proprioceptive afferent fibers for coordinated reflexes of the eyes, neck, and body for maintaining equilibrium in accordance with the posture and movement of the head.

THE VESTIBULAR NERVE AND ITS CENTRAL CONNECTIONS

There are three semicircular canals—the anterior, lateral (horizontal), and posterior—which are roughly arranged in three planes of space at right angles to one another. Receptors in the semicircular canals respond to rotatory movement (angular acceleration and deceleration), which evokes movement of endolymphatic fluid and deflection of hairs of the sensory epithelium. The utriculus responds to gravitational forces and to linear acceleration, chiefly in the horizontal plane. The sacculi respond to vibrational stimuli and to linear acceleration in the dorsoventral plane. Axons of bipolar cells of the vestibular ganglion pass through the internal auditory canal and reach the upper medulla in company with the cochlear nerve. Most of the fibers of the vestibular nerve bifurcate into ascending and descending branches and terminate in the vestibular nuclei, which are clustered in the lateral part of the floor of the fourth ventricle (Fig. 37): the *medial vestibular nucleus* (of Schwalbe), the *lateral vestibular nucleus* (of Deiter), the *superior vestibular nucleus* (of Bechterew), and the *inferior vestibular* nucleus (descending spinal). The afferent fibers innervating the cristae of the semicircular canals terminate primarily in the medial and superior vestibular nuclei. The afferent fibers innervating the maculae of the utricle and saccule terminate in the lateral, inferior and medial vestibular nuclei.

A few primary fibers of the vestibular nerve pass directly to the cerebellum, ending in the cortex of the flocculonodular lobe. Connections are made within the cerebellum to the *nucleus fastigii,* which gives rise to the *fastigiobulbar tract* (tract of Russell). The fibers of this tract are crossed and uncrossed and terminate in all of the vestibular nuclei and in the reticular formation of the pons and medulla. As they pass from the cerebellum, they loop around the superior cerebellar peduncle to form the *uncinate fasciculus* (hook bundle). Other fibers from the fastigial nucleus, which are uncrossed, pass from the cerebellum on the medial side of the inferior cerebellar peduncle and constitute a portion of the peduncle sometimes referred to as the *juxtarestiform* body. The fibers of the juxtarestiform body terminate in the vestibular nuclei and in the reticular formation.

THE VESTIBULOSPINAL TRACTS

Two vestibulospinal tracts arise from the vestibular nuclei. The lateral tract, which is uncrossed, comes from the lateral vestibular nucleus; the medial tract, which is primarily uncrossed, comes chiefly from the medial vestibular nucleus. The *lateral vestibulospinal tract* extends to the sacral level of the cord. The *medial vestibulospinal tract* extends through the cervical level. Both tracts terminate along their course almost exclusively upon interneurons in laminae VII and VIII, which in turn synapse upon alpha and gamma lower motoneurons (see Chapter 4). Impulses descending in these tracts assist the local myotatic reflexes and reinforce the tonus of the extensor muscles of the trunk and limbs, producing enough extra force to support the body against gravity and maintain an upright posture.

An animal whose brain stem has been transected at the midbrain level develops a condition known as *decerebrate rigidity.* This condition is characterized by marked rigidity of the extensor muscles of all the limbs as well as the trunk and neck. Decerebrate rigidity occurs in humans and, in this case, the limbs are all extended with the arms adducted and internally rotated at the shoulders. Decerebrate rigidity results from a marked tonic enhancement of activity descending from the brain stem through the vestibulospinal and reticulospinal tracts, which exert a strong excitatory influence upon muscle tone, particularly in extensor muscles. Normally, muscle tone is maintained by a balance of inhibitory and facilitatory activity descending from the cerebral hemispheres to the level of the spinal cord. Removal of the influence of the cerebral hemispheres by transection of the brain stem allows excessive activity in the vestibulospinal and reticulospinal

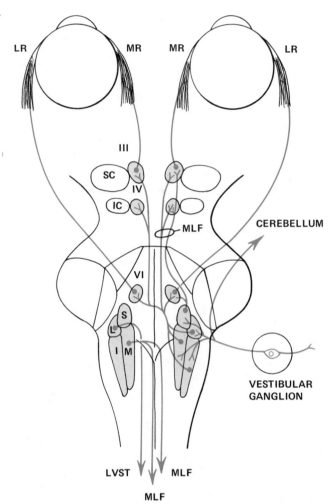

FIGURE 37. Major pathways arising from the vestibular nuclei. On the left side of the diagram the descending pathways are illustrated; on the right side, those ascending fibers that enter the medial longitudinal fasciculus and control vestibularly mediated eye movements. Only the connections to the medial and lateral rectus muscles, controlling horizontal gaze, are shown. I = inferior vestibular nucleus; IC = inferior colliculus; L = lateral vestibular nucleus; LR = lateral rectus muscle; LVST = lateral vestibulospinal tract; M = medial vestibular nucleus; MLF = medial longitudinal fasciculus; MR = medial rectus muscle; S = superior vestibular nucleus; SC = superior colliculus; III = oculomotor nucleus; IV = trochlear nucleus; VI = abducens nucleus.

tracts to occur without control. At the spinal level, decerebrate rigidity results from a marked tonic facilitation of gamma motoneuron activity, which increases the rate of firing of muscle spindle afferents and, in turn, increases the firing of alpha motoneurons to extensor muscles. Decerebrate rigidity is abolished by transection of the dorsal roots because this interrupts the gamma motoneuron–spindle afferent reflex arc. Decerebrate rigidity is abolished also by lesions of the central nervous system that interrupt the descending vestibular and reticular pathways.

THE VESTIBULO-OCULAR PATHWAYS

The vestibular system is extremely important in controlling _conjugate eye movements_ reflexly in response to head movement and to the position of the head in space. Fibers from the superior, medial, and to a lesser extent, the lateral and inferior vestibular nuclei project rostrally in the _medial longitudinal fasciculus_ (MLF). The projections from the superior nucleus are uncrossed, while those from the other vestibular nuclei are both crossed and uncrossed. The fibers synapse on the somatic motor nuclei of the cranial nerves (_abducens_, VI; _trochlear_, IV; and _oculomotor_, III) that supply the extraocular muscles. Other fibers from the MLF, which indirectly may influence eye movements, project to several small nuclear groups located in the vicinity of the oculomotor nuclear complex and the pretectal area. These include the interstitial nucleus of Cajal, the nucleus of Darkschewitsch, the nucleus of the posterior commissure, and possibly the thalamic nuclei.

Vestibular reflexes, in cooperation with certain reflexes of the optic system, enable the eyes to remain fixed on stationary objects while the head and body are moving. Turning the head slightly to the right causes a small flow of endolymph in the horizontal semicircular canals. The flow is directed to the left because the fluid's inertia makes it lag behind the movement of the head. The flow of endolymph causes neural activity to pass from receptors in the ampulla of the horizontal semicircular canals to the vestibular nuclei. From there the activity passes through the MLF to excite the left abducens nucleus (to innervate the left lateral rectus muscle) and to the right oculomotor nucleus (to innervate the right medial rectus muscle) (see Fig. 37). Simultaneously, activity in the MLF inhibits the innervation to the left medial rectus and the right lateral rectus muscles. As a result, the eyes are turned the proper distance to the left to keep the fields of vision unchanged.

TESTS OF VESTIBULAR FUNCTION

If stimulation of hair cells in the appropriate ampulla of the semicircular canal is persistent, the eyes draw slowly to one side until they reach a limit and then jerk quickly to the opposite side. These movements are repeated in rapid succession, producing tremorlike oscillations of the eyes, known as nystagmus. The *direction of nystagmus* is designated according to the direction of the *fast component*, although this is opposite to the movement induced by stimulation from the semicircular canal. The fact that vestibular stimulation evokes nystagmus provides a basis for clinical tests of vestibular function.

A *rotation test* of vestibular function may be performed by whirling the subject in a revolving chair with the head tilted forward 30 degrees to bring the horizontal canals parallel with the floor. Movement is stopped abruptly after 10 or 12 turns. Momentum causes the endolymph to continue to flow in the direction in which the head had been turning, even though the head is now stationary. The induced nystagmus lasts about 30 seconds in normal individuals. If rotation has been to the left, endolymph flows to the left, and the slow component of the nystagmus is to the left. Since the quick component is to the right, it is called "nystagmus to the right." With a special chair designed to rotate the subject's head in any plane, it is possible to test each of the three pairs of semicircular canals individually. The orientation of the canals is such that the two horizontal canals are one pair; the right anterior and left posterior canals are in the same plane and constitute the second pair; and the right posterior and left anterior canals are the third pair.

Caloric, or *thermal, tests* of nystagmus permit the vestibular system of each side to be tested separately. The subject is usually seated with the head tilted backward about 60 degrees to bring the horizontal semicircular canal into a vertical plane, then the external auditory canal is irrigated with cold or warm water. Warm water raises the temperature of the endolymph in the semicircular canal and causes it to rise. Stimulation of hair cells by the current flowing past the ampulla produces nystagmus. With warm water in the right ear, the current going up produces a flow equivalent to flow to the left in the horizontal position. Thus the nystagmus has its slow component to the left and its quick component to the right. If cold water is used, the current is reversed and nystagmus is in the opposite direction.

Irritation or destruction of the vestibule, vestibular nerve, or vestibular nuclei commonly produces nystagmus and may also cause deviation of the eyes to one side. If the right vestibular nerve is severed, the influence of the remaining left vestibular apparatus is unbalanced and causes nystagmus with the slow component to the right and conjugate deviation of the eyes to the right. In a few weeks, this effect is overcome by the compensating influence of voluntary and visual reflex circuits. The quick component of nystagmus produced by an irritative lesion is usually toward the side of the lesion, but at times it may be difficult to distinguish effects of irritation on one side from those of destruction on the other. Although *horizontal nystagmus* is the most common type, vertical or rotatory forms of nystagmus also occur. Nystagmus results from lesions of the vestibular system, including its peripheral and central connections, and also from lesions of the brain stem and cerebellum. Nystagmus can result from chronic visual impairment and from a number of toxic substances.

SENSORY ASPECTS
OF VESTIBULAR STIMULATION

Stimulation of the vestibular apparatus, whether by motion of the body or by artificial means, produces definite conscious effects which take the form of a false sense of motion. Vertigo is a sensation of whirling. The individual may have a feeling that his body is rotating, or it may seem to him that external objects are spinning around. Feelings of giddiness, faintness, and lightheadedness may be vaguely described in somewhat similar terms, but they should not be mistaken for true vertigo. Menière's disease is a condition characterized by sudden attacks of severe vertigo, usually associated with unilateral deafness and tinnitus, and with nausea, vomiting, and prostration. Edema with increased pressure of fluid in the labyrinth is thought to be responsible for this condition. Motion sickness during travel by air or sea is a familiar manifestation of prolonged and unusual stimulation of the vestibular apparatus.

15

THE CEREBELLUM

The cerebellum is situated in the posterior cranial fossa. It is attached to the medulla, pons, and midbrain by the cerebellar peduncles that lie at the sides of the fourth ventricle on the ventral aspect of the cerebellum. The tentorium cerebelli, a transverse fold of the dura mater, stretches horizontally over the superior surface of the cerebellum and separates it from the overlying occipital lobes of the cerebrum. The surface of the cerebellum is corrugated by numerous parallel folds known as folia. A layer of gray matter, the cerebellar cortex, covers the surface and encloses an internal core of white matter. Four pairs of *deep cerebellar nuclei* are buried within the cerebellum. From medial to lateral these consist of the *fastigial, globose, emboliform,* and *dentate nuclei.* The globose and emboliform nuclei commonly are grouped together and termed the *interposed nuclei.*

PRIMARY SUBDIVISIONS OF THE CEREBELLUM

The cerebellum is divided into two large lateral masses, the *cerebellar hemispheres,* which fuse near the midline with a narrow middle portion called the *vermis.* There are three major anatomic components to the cerebellum:

1. The *flocculonodular lobe* consists of the paired flocculi, which are small appendages in the posterior inferior region, and the nodulus,

which is the inferior part of the vermis. This portion of the cerebellum is also termed the *archicerebellum* since phylogenetically it is the oldest part of the structure.

2. The *anterior lobe*, of modest size, is the portion of the cerebellum that lies anterior to the primary fissure. This lobe corresponds approximately to the *paleocerebellum*, which is the second oldest part of the cerebellum phylogenetically.

3. The *posterior lobe* is the largest part of the cerebellum and is located between the other two lobes. It contains the major portions of the cerebellar hemispheres and is known as the *neocerebellum*.

The flocculonodular lobe receives projections heavily from the vestibular nuclei. The anterior lobe, particularly its vermal portion, receives input from the spinocerebellar pathways. The flocculonodular and anterior lobes are the predominant regions of the cerebellum in primitive vertebrates. The posterior lobe receives projections from the cerebral hemispheres and has become greatly expanded in mammals that have developed an extensive cerebral cortex.

The foregoing description presents the *transverse arrangement* of the cerebellum. This is based upon the formation of 10 rostrocaudally arranged lobules during embryologic development and the formation of various transverse fissures. Currently, a more functionally useful method of describing the cerebellum is based upon *longitudinal sagittal zonal patterns.* This classification subdivides each half of the cerebellum into three mediolaterally arranged longitudinal strips, including cerebellar cortex, underlying white matter, and deep cerebellar nuclei: (1) the vermal region with the fastigial nuclei; (2) the paravermal region with the interposed nuclei; and (3) the lateral (hemispheric) region with the dentate nuclei.

The Cerebellar Cortex

The cerebellar cortex consists of three layers (Fig. 38):

1. The *molecular layer* (outermost), containing two types of neurons, the *stellate* and *basket cells,* dendrites of Purkinje and Golgi type II cells, and axons (T-shaped parallel fibers) of the granule cells.

2. The *Purkinje cell layer* (middle), containing the cell bodies of Purkinje cells, which are very large, flasklike neurons that have enormous dendritic arborizations extending up into the molecular layer, and long axons that synapse either upon deep cerebellar nuclei or vestibular nuclei. Collaterals of Purkinje cell axons make synaptic contact with Golgi cells, other Purkinje cells, basket cells, and stellate cells.

3. The *granular layer* (innermost), containing numerous *granule cells* (neurons), *Golgi type II cells* (neurons), and *glomeruli* (complex syn-

aptic nodules that contain axons of incoming mossy fibers, axons and dendrites of Golgi type II cells, and dendrites of granule cells). Each glomerulus is encased in glial cells.

The relationships between the various neurons of the cerebellar cortex are quite complex, and a discussion of these is beyond the scope of this book. However, a few important features are essential to an understanding of how the cerebellum functions.

Afferents to the cerebellum terminate either in the granule cell layer (in the glomeruli) as *mossy fibers* or upon the dendrites of Purkinje cells as *climbing fibers*. Mossy fiber afferents are derived from the spinal cord, pon-

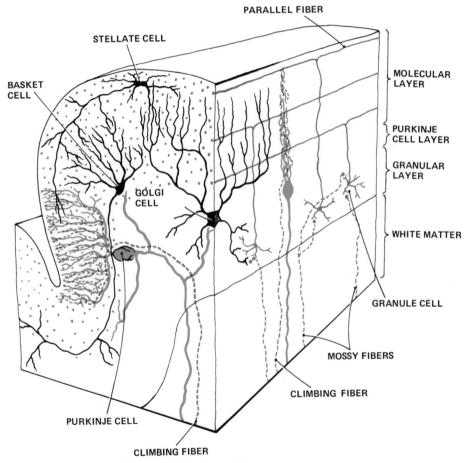

FIGURE 38. The cerebellar cortex in perspective.

tine nuclei, vestibular receptors and nuclei, trigeminal nuclei, reticular nuclei, and deep cerebellar nuclei. Climbing fiber afferents are thought to be derived exclusively from the olive. Both mossy fiber and climbing fiber inputs are excitatory. Excited granule cells, through their axonal processes (parallel fibers) can excite Purkinje cells, basket cells, stellate cells, and Golgi type II cells. In turn, the basket and stellate cells inhibit Purkinje and Golgi type II cells. The Golgi type II cells inhibit granule cells. Finally, *the Purkinje cells (the only route for all information exiting from the cerebellar cortex) are inhibitory to the deep cerebellar and vestibular nuclei. Consequently, of all the neurons whose cells reside within the cerebellar cortex, the granule cell is the only excitatory one.*

Afferents to the cerebellum also originate in the locus ceruleus and in the raphe nuclei of the brain stem. The afferents from the locus ceruleus are noradrenergic and terminate in the deep cerebellar nuclei, the granular layer, and the Purkinje cell layer. The afferents from the raphe nuclei are serotonergic and terminate in the deep cerebellar nuclei, the granular layer, and the molecular layer.

The Peduncles of the Cerebellum

The three paired cerebellar peduncles are composed of large numbers of fibers entering and leaving the cerebellum to connect it with other parts of the nervous system.

The *inferior cerebellar peduncle* (restiform body) consists chiefly of afferent fibers. The peduncle contains a single efferent tract, the fastigiobulbar tract, which goes to the vestibular nuclei and completes a vestibular circuit through the cerebellum. Afferent fibers enter the inferior cerebellar peduncle from at least six sources (Fig. 39): (1) fibers from the vestibular nerve and nuclei; (2) olivocerebellar fibers from the inferior olivary nuclei; (3) the dorsal spinocerebellar tract; (4) some of the fibers from the rostral spinocerebellar tract; (5) the cuneocerebellar tract from the main and external cuneate nuclei in the medulla; and (6) reticulocerebellar fibers.

The *middle cerebellar peduncle* (brachium pontis) consists almost entirely of crossed afferent fibers from the pontine nuclei in the gray substance of the basal part of the pons (pontocerebellar or transverse pontine fibers). The major projections to the pontine nuclei originate within the cerebral cortex.

The *superior cerebellar peduncle* (brachium conjunctivum) consists principally of efferent projections from the cerebellum. Rubral, thalamic, and reticular projections arise from the dentate and interposed nuclei. The fastigiobulbar tract also runs with the superior peduncle for a short distance before it enters the inferior cerebellar peduncle. The superior cerebellar peduncle contains afferent projections from the ventral spinocerebellar tract, a portion of the rostral spinocerebellar tract, and trigeminocerebellar projections.

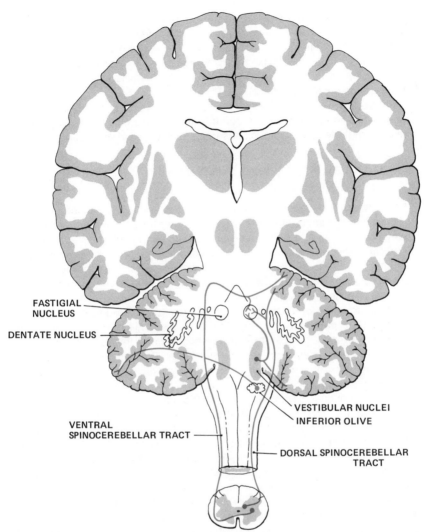

FIGURE 39. The central nervous system connections of the dorsal and ventral spinocerebellar tracts, the fastigial nuclei, and the vestibular nuclei.

FUNCTIONS OF THE CEREBELLUM

The cerebellum participates with other central nervous system structures in the execution of a wide variety of movements. It is needed to maintain the proper posture and balance for walking and running; to execute sequential movements for eating, dressing, and writing; to participate in rapidly alternating repetitive movements and in smooth pursuit movements; and to control certain properties of movements, including trajectory, velocity, and acceleration. Voluntary movements can proceed without assistance from the cerebellum, but such movements are clumsy and disorganized. Lack of motor skill as a result of cerebellar dysfunction is called *dyssynergia* (also *asynergia* or *cerebellar ataxia*).

Although the cerebellum receives large numbers of afferent fibers, conscious perception does not occur in the cerebellum, nor do its efferent fibers contribute to conscious sensations elsewhere in the brain.

Afferent and Efferent Pathways of the Cerebellum

The cortex of the cerebellum and the deep cerebellar nuclei are furnished with a constant account of the progress of motor activity by signals from many sources. First, it is informed of the commands being issued from the cerebral cortex by a flow of nerve impulses through three cerebrocerebellar projection pathways. The largest of these is the corticopontocerebellar pathway, which is a crossed path connecting one cerebral hemisphere with the cerebellar hemisphere on the opposite side by way of the *corticopontine tract* and the *pontocerebellar projections* that ascend through the *middle cerebellar peduncle* (Fig. 40). The other pathways originate primarily in the motor areas of the cerebral cortex and include the *cerebro-olivocerebellar* and *cerebroreticulocerebellar* pathways. Further communication received by the cerebellar cortex consists of a stream of information from the skin, joints, and muscles of the limbs and trunk of the body, mediated by the spinocerebellar tracts. All sensory modalities, including tactile, auditory, vestibular, and visual, reach the cerebellum. These messages enter a vast pool of cerebellar cortical neurons where integrations take place. In general, the vermis of the anterior lobe and parts of the posterior lobe receive afferent input from the spinal cord, the flocculonodular lobe receives a major projection from the vestibular system, and the cerebellar hemispheres receive their major input from the cerebral cortex.

Afferent input from essentially all sources reaches both the deep cerebellar nuclei and the cerebellar cortex. The result is an increase in excitability of the deep nuclei and the Purkinje cells of the cerebellar cortex. The Purkinje cells provide strong inhibitory control over neurons of the deep nuclei. At present, it appears that the inhibitory control of the Purkinje cell over the excitability of the deep cerebellar nuclei is a key aspect of cerebellar function. Through interactions between the cerebellar cortex and the deep nuclei, the cerebellum is able to provide appropriate corrections to ensure that the speed and accuracy of movements will be adequate for each task being undertaken by the motor system.

The efferent pathways by which the cerebellum is able to influence movement are best understood by examining the projections of the deep cerebellar nuclei. The fastigial nucleus sends projections to the reticular

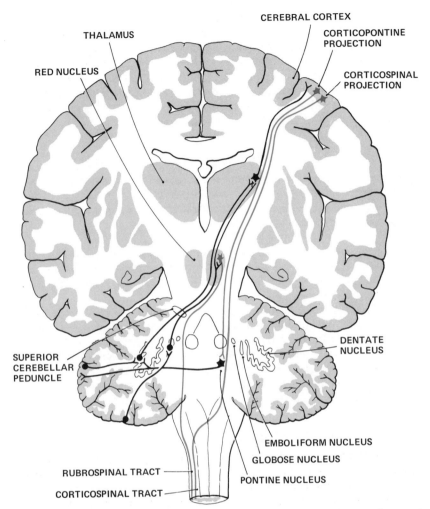

FIGURE 40. The central nervous system connections of the dentate nucleus and interposed (emboliform and globose) nuclei.

and vestibular nuclei of the brain stem. These nuclei, in turn, send projections into the spinal cord and are concerned with posture and balance. The interposed nuclei of each side of the cerebellum send projections through the superior cerebellar peduncle to the red nucleus of the contralateral side. The red nucleus, in turn, gives rise to axons of the rubrospinal tract (Fig. 40). This projection crosses the midline and projects into the spinal cord. Thus the origin of this pathway in the interposed nuclei and the terminal portion are on the same side of the body. Projections from both the dentate and the interposed nuclei exit through the superior cerebellar peduncle to the contralateral ventrolateral nucleus of the thalamus. Thalamo-cortical fibers from the ventrolateral nucleus relay impulses to the motor regions of the ipsilateral frontal lobe. The thalamocortical projections in the frontal lobe make contact with cortical efferent fibers that pass through the pyramidal tract and make connection with the contralateral side of the spinal cord through the corticospinal pathway. Thus the origin of this pathway in the dentate and interposed nuclei and its termination in the spinal cord are on the same side of the body (see Fig. 40).

Feedback Circuits Through the Cerebellum

The general scheme of operation of the cerebellum allows nerve impulses to be returned, or fed back, to the same region from which they originated. Briefly, the following are important feedback circuits involving the cerebellum:

1. The vermal region receives information from the spinal cord and sends back information indirectly by the fastigial nucleus through the reticular formation (reticulospinal tracts) and vestibular nuclei (vestibulospinal tracts) to the cord.
2. The flocculonodular lobe receives information from the vestibular system and returns information through fastigiobulbar and fastigioreticulovestibular pathways.
3. The lateral (hemisphere) region receives information from the cerebral cortex and sends information back through the dentatothalamocortical path to exert an influence on the cerebrum and through the corticospinal tract to influence the spinal cord.

Clinical Signs of Cerebellar Dysfunction

From the clinical perspective, the cerebellum is organized into a series of sagittal zones. The clinical signs of cerebellar dysfunction can be separated into those resulting from disease of the midline zone of the cerebellum and those resulting from disease of the lateral portions.

DISEASE OF THE MIDLINE ZONE OF THE CEREBELLUM

The midline zone of the cerebellum consists of the anterior and posterior vermis, the flocculonodular lobe, and the fastigial nuclei. Disease of these regions produces:

1. *Disorders of stance and gait.* The stance is usually on a broad base with the feet several inches apart. There may be a severe truncal tremor. It is difficult for the patient to walk in tandem, placing the heel of one foot directly in front of the toes of the other foot.

2. *Titubation.* This is a rhythmic tremor of the body or head occurring several times per second.
3. *Rotated or tilted postures of the head.* The head may be maintained, rotated, or tilted to the left or right. The side of the deviation does not usually indicate the site of the cerebellar disease.
4. *Ocular motor disorders.* A number of disturbances of ocular function result from cerebellar disease, the most prominent of which is nystagmus. This consists of rhythmical oscillatory movements of one or both eyes occurring with the eyes gazing straight ahead or with ocular deviation.

DISEASE OF THE LATERAL (HEMISPHERIC) ZONE OF THE CEREBELLUM

For clinical purposes, the lateral cerebellar zone consists of the cerebellar hemisphere and the dentate and interposed nuclei of each side. Disease of this region produces:

1. *Hypotonia.* This is a decrease in the resistance to passive manipulation of the limbs, appearing in one or several limbs at the time of cerebellar injury. It often decreases with time. It is detected clinically by manipulating the limbs about the joints and not by palpating the muscles.
2. *Dysarthria.* In cerebellar disease speech may be slow, slurred, and labored, but comprehension remains intact and grammar does not suffer.
3. *Dysmetria.* This is a disturbance of the trajectory or placement of a body part during active movements. The limb may fall short of its goal in hypometria, or it may extend beyond its goal in hypermetria.
4. *Dysdiadochokinesis and dysrhythmokinesis.* Dysdiadochokinesis is a manifestation of the decomposition of movements in cerebellar disease, demonstrated by testing alternating or fine repetitive movements. Dysrhythmokinesis is a disorder of the rhythm of rapidly alternating movements. It can be evoked by asking the patient to tap out a rhythm such as three rapid beats followed by one delayed beat. In cerebellar disease, the rhythm of the movement is disturbed.
5. *Ataxia.* This term describes comprehensively the various problems of movement resulting chiefly from the combined effects of dysmetria and decomposition of movement. There are errors in the sequence and speed of the components of each movement. An ataxia of gait results in a veering of the path from side to side with difficulty walking in a straight line.
6. *Tremor.* Cerebellar disease results in static and kinetic tremors. Static tremor is demonstrated by asking the patient to extend the

arms parallel to the floor with the hands open. A rhythmic oscillation generated at the shoulder will be seen. A kinetic tremor can be brought out by having the patient alternately touch his nose and then touch the examiner's finger, which is held at a full arm's length away from the patient. It can be tested also by asking the patient to place the heel of one foot on the knee of the opposite leg and run the heel down the shin. These movements result in a side-to-side coarse tremor, which is generated at the proximal joints (shoulder and hip).

7. *Ocular motor disorders.* A number of disorders of eye movement result from injury to the cerebellar hemispheres. The most common disorder is nystagmus.

Cerebellar defects are offset, to a considerable extent, by other mechanisms in the brain if sufficient time is given. Consequently, symptoms are less severe in slowly progressive disease processes than in acute injuries to the cerebellum.

Somatotopic localization of separate body regions in the cerebellar cortex has been demonstrated in experimental animals. These studies have revealed an extremely complex representation of body parts. Despite the complexity of the organization of the cerebellum, however, it is clear that the right side of the body is under the influence of the right cerebellar hemisphere and that any symptoms that occur unilaterally are found on the same side as the lesion in the cerebellum. This contrasts strikingly with cerebral lesions that produce contralateral effects.

16

LESIONS OF THE BRAIN STEM

Since the brain stem contains a compact arrangement of diverse structures, a single lesion commonly damages several of them simultaneously. The structures frequently injured are (1) the afferent or efferent components of the cranial nerve nuclei, which innervate structures on the ipsilateral side of the body, and (2) the long descending motor and long ascending sensory pathways, both of which innervate structures on the contralateral side of the body. As a consequence of this anatomic arrangement, a unilateral lesion of the brain stem often causes loss of function of one or more cranial nerves on the ipsilateral side of the body and a hemiplegia with a hemisensory loss on the contralateral side. Brain stem lesions result from diverse types of pathology, including hemorrhages, vascular occlusions, tumors, and lesions of multiple sclerosis. Many of the resulting clinical disorders have been given eponyms, but since there is considerable lack of uniformity in their usage, only the more familiar ones will be discussed.

contra hemiplegia

LESIONS OF THE BASAL PART OF THE MEDULLA

Several of the individual cranial nerves pass close to the pyramidal tract before they emerge from the brain stem. A single lesion that includes the nerve and the tract at this point produces loss of function of the cranial nerve on the side of the lesion and a contralateral hemiplegia. For example, a lesion of the right hypoglossal nerve and the right pyramid results in paralysis of the muscles of the right half of the tongue together with left hemiplegia (Fig. 41, lesion 1). The paralysis of the arm and leg is on the side opposite the lesion because the pyramidal tract crosses to the left caudal to the site of the lesion, at the junction of the medulla with the cervical spinal cord. If the lesion occurs acutely, as with a vascular occlusion, the arm and leg show a hypotonic paralysis, with weakness, diminished resistance to passive manipulation, decreased deep tendon (muscle stretch) reflexes, loss of superficial reflexes, and absence of the response to plantar stimulation. Within a month to six weeks after an acute lesion, or with a chronic lesion, the arm and leg develop a spastic paralysis, with weakness, "clasp-knife" resistance to passive manipulation, hyperreflexia, loss of superficial reflexes, and an extensor plantar (Babinski) response. The tongue deviates to the right side when protruded and, progressively the right half of the tongue becomes atrophic.

An extension of this lesion across the midline may damage the left pyramid and produce additional signs of upper motoneuron involvement in

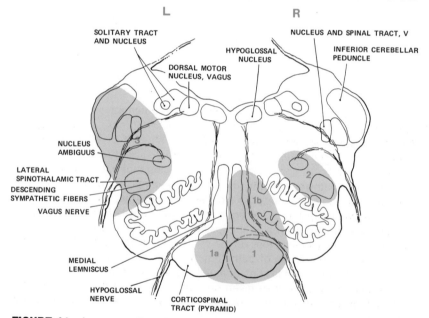

FIGURE 41. A cross section of the medulla. The shaded areas show the positions of lesions. *1.* A lesion of the right hypoglossal nerve and right pyramid. *1a.* An extension of the lesion involving the left pyramid. *2.* A lesion of the nucleus ambiguus and lateral spinothalamic tract. *3.* A lesion affecting the dorsolateral portion of the medulla, involving the inferior cerebellar peduncle, the spinal tract and nucleus of the trigeminal nerve, the lateral spinothalamic tract, the nucleus ambiguus, the vestibular nuclei, the descending sympathetic pathways, and the emerging fibers of the vagus and glossopharyngeal nerves.

the right extremities (Fig. 41, lesion 1a). If the same lesion is enlarged in the dorsal direction, it will affect the right medial lemniscus, and defects will occur in position sense, vibration sense, and tactile discrimination (Fig. 41, lesion 1b). Since the fibers of the medial lemniscus cross in the lower part of the medulla caudal to this level, the sensory signs will appear on the left side of the body.

LESIONS OF THE CENTRAL REGION OF THE UPPER MEDULLA

A small lesion in the lateral part of the reticular formation of the upper medulla may include the nucleus ambiguus and the lateral spinothalamic tract simultaneously (Fig. 41, lesion 2). When the lesion is on the right side, it causes a loss of pain and temperature sense on the left side of the body, except for the face. The sensory effects are contralateral because fibers of the lateral spinothalamic tract are crossed near their origin. Destruction of the nucleus ambiguus paralyzes the voluntary muscles in the pharynx and larynx supplied by the right vagus and glossopharyngeal nerves. Failure of the right side of the soft palate to contract causes difficulty in swallowing and, on phonation, the palate and uvula are drawn to the nonparalyzed left side. Loss of function of the right vocal cord results in hoarseness of the voice.

A larger lesion in the central region of the upper medulla may extend to the medial lemniscus and to the solitary tract. Interrupting the fibers of the lemniscus on the right causes the additional loss of vibration sense, position sense, and tactile discrimination on the left. Destruction of the solitary tract results in anesthesia of the mucosa of the right side of the pharynx and loss of taste sensations on the right side of the tongue.

LESIONS OF THE DORSOLATERAL REGION OF THE UPPER MEDULLA (WALLENBERG'S SYNDROME)

The posterior inferior cerebellar artery, a branch of the vertebral artery, supplies the dorsolateral portion of the medulla and the inferior surface of the cerebellar vermis. A lesion in this position is commonly the result of arterial occlusion by thrombosis of the posterior inferior cerebellar artery or the vertebral artery. The damage involves the inferior cerebellar peduncle, the spinal tract and nucleus of the trigeminal nerve, the lateral spinothalamic tract, the nucleus ambiguus, the descending sympathetic pathways, and the emerging fibers of the vagus and glossopharyngeal nerves (Fig. 41, lesion 3). The vestibular nuclei often are affected as well. Loss of function of the spinocerebellar fibers in the inferior cerebellar peduncle results in cerebellar dyssynergia and hypotonia on the side of the lesion. Injury to the spinal tract of the trigeminal nerve causes loss of the sensations of pain and temperature from the ipsilateral side of the face and loss of the ipsilateral corneal reflex, while damage to the lateral spinothalamic tract is responsible for loss of pain and temperature sense in the limbs and trunk of the side opposite to the lesion. Damage to the vestibular nuclei causes nystagmus. Injury of the descending sympathetic pathways results in an ipsilateral Horner's syndrome, with pupillary constriction, ptosis, enophthalmos, and loss of sweating in half of the face. Loss of function of the nucleus ambiguus and the fibers of IX and X leads to paralysis of the soft palate, pharynx, and larynx with dysphagia and dysphonia.

LESIONS OF THE BASAL PORTION OF THE CAUDAL PART OF THE PONS

A lesion so placed that it includes the right corticospinal tract and the emerging fibers of the right abducens nerve results in an ipsilateral abducens palsy and a contralateral hemiplegia (Fig. 42, lesion 1). In the patient with a chronic lesion, an upper motoneuron type of paralysis of the left arm and leg will be observed, as well as an internal deviation of the right eye due to paralysis of the lateral rectus and the unopposed pull of the medial rectus muscle.

Lesions of this part of the brain stem often extend far enough laterally to include fibers of the facial nerve and thus also produce a peripheral type of facial paralysis. When the facial nerve is included, the condition is sometimes called the *Millard-Gubler syndrome* (Fig. 42, lesion 1a).

A similar lesion with considerable dorsal expansion into the pontine tegmentum will involve the right medial lemniscus, the paramedian pontine reticular formation, and the right medial longitudinal fasciculus (Fig. 42, lesion 1b). The effect of interrupting fibers of the medial lemniscus is loss of position sense, vibration sense, and tactile discrimination on the left side of the body. Damage to the neurons responsible for conjugate lateral gaze in the paramedian pontine reticular formation abolishes the ability to turn the eyes voluntarily to the right, resulting in paralysis of right lateral gaze. The eyes may be drawn to the left by the predominating influence of the nonparalyzed antagonistic muscles, but such an effect is temporary. The combination of symptoms produced by this lesion is known as Foville's syndrome.

Damage to the medial longitudinal fasciculus bilaterally results in internuclear ophthalmoplegia, a disorder commonly found in multiple sclerosis. With attempted gaze to one side, the adduction fails to move beyond the midline, and coarse nystagmus develops in the abducting eye. The same abnormality develops with gaze to the opposite side. Despite loss of adduction on attempted lateral gaze, convergence often is preserved.

LESIONS OF THE CEREBELLOPONTINE ANGLE

An acoustic neuroma is a slowly growing tumor that arises from Schwann cells in the sheath of the acoustic nerve close to the attachment of the

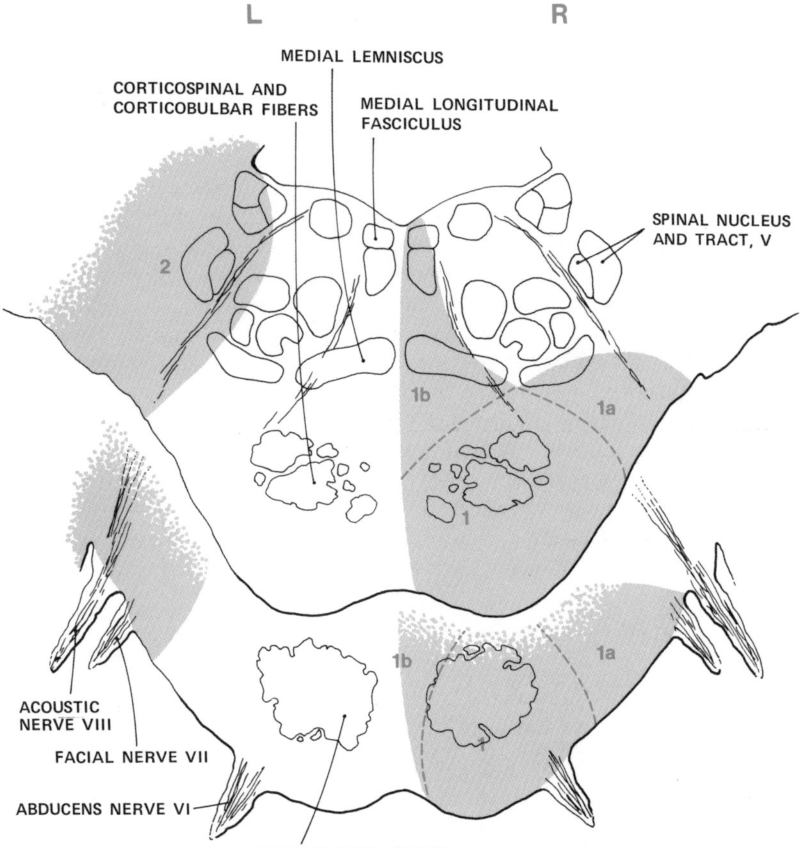

FIGURE 42. A cross section of the caudal portion of the pons. The shaded areas indicate the positions of lesions. *1.* A lesion of the right corticospinal tract and the emerging fibers of the right abducens nerve. *1A.* An extension of this lesion to include the facial nerve. *1B.* An extension of this lesion into the pontine tegmentum, involving the right medial lemniscus and right medial longitudinal fasciculus. *2.* The region affected by a cerebellopontine angle tumor.

nerve to the brain stem. The tumor exerts pressure on the lateral region of the caudal part of the pons near the cerebellopontine angle (Fig. 42, lesion 2). At first the symptoms are those of eighth nerve damage. Progressive deafness will be noted, as well as absence of normal labyrinthine (vestibular) responses and, sometimes, horizontal nystagmus. Later, cerebellar dyssynergia appears on the side of the lesion due to compression of the cerebellar peduncles. If the tumor becomes extremely large, damage to the spinal tract and nucleus of the fifth nerve can occur, abolishing the corneal reflex and causing diminished pain and temperature sensibility over the face on the side of the injury. A peripheral type of facial paralysis, also on the side of the lesion, can result from damage to the fibers of the seventh nerve.

LESIONS OF THE MIDDLE REGION OF THE PONS

A large lesion in the basal part of the right side of the pons can affect the right corticospinal tract and the emerging fibers of the right trigeminal nerve to produce an ipsilateral fifth nerve palsy and a contralateral hemiplegia (Fig. 43, lesion 1). Involvement of the motor fibers of the fifth nerve leads to paralysis of the muscles of the right side of the jaw so that, when the mouth is opened, the jaw deviates to the right. Damage to the sensory fibers of the fifth nerve causes anesthesia of the right side of the face with loss of the right corneal reflex. In the patient with a chronic lesion there is an upper motoneuron paralysis of the left arm and leg.

A lesion in the same region that extends further upward will enter the tegmentum of the pons and destroy the medial lemniscus. This results in loss of position sense, vibration sense, and tactile discrimination on the left side of the body. A lesion in this location also interrupts the small number of aberrant uncrossed fibers of the corticobulbar and corticotectal tracts that

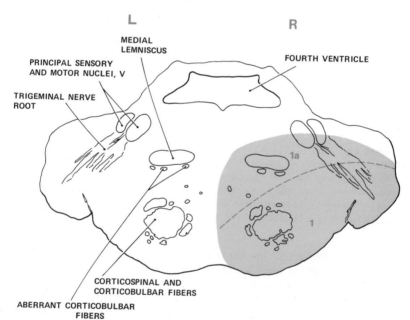

FIGURE 43. A cross section of the middle region of the pons. The shaded areas indicate the positions of lesions. *1.* A lesion affecting the right corticospinal tract and the emerging fibers of the right trigeminal nerve. *1A.* An extension of this lesion to involve the medial lemniscus and the corticobulbar tract.

have separated from the corticospinal tracts and, in this region, lie near the medial lemniscus (Fig. 43, lesion 1a). In addition to left hemiplegia there is paralysis of the superficial muscles of the lower part of the left side of the face, the left side of the soft palate, and the left half of the tongue due to interruption of upper motor neuron fibers to the motor nuclei of the seventh, tenth, and twelfth cranial nerves. The lesion also destroys the tectal projections to the paramedian pontine reticular formation before they cross, interrupting the pathway from the right frontal lobe that produces voluntary turning of the eyes to the left. This results in paralysis of left lateral gaze and deviation of the eyes tonically to the right.

LESIONS OF THE BASAL PART OF THE MIDBRAIN (WEBER'S SYNDROME)

A lesion of the right cerebral peduncle and the right oculomotor nerve produces left hemiplegia combined with external strabismus of the right eye and loss of the ability to raise the right upper eyelid. The eye cannot be adducted beyond the midline, and it cannot be elevated or lowered. The right pupil is dilated because of interruption of the parasympathetic fibers in the third nerve. The corticobulbar tract may not be affected, since many of its fibers diverge from the corticospinal tract at this level and shift to a more dorsal position as they continue downward. If the lesion extends dorsally, however, it may include most of these fibers and cause weakness of the face, soft palate, and tongue contralateral to the lesion. In this instance there will be weakness of the muscles of the lower part of the left side of the face, the soft palate and uvula will be drawn to the right, and the tongue will deviate to the left when protruded (Fig. 44, lesion 1).

LESIONS OF THE TEGMENTUM OF THE MIDBRAIN (BENEDIKT'S SYNDROME)

A lesion of the tegmentum of the midbrain affects the fibers of the oculomotor nerve, the medial lemniscus, the red nucleus, and fibers of the superior cerebellar peduncle (Fig. 44, lesion 2). If the lesion is located on the left side, loss of function of the left oculomotor nerve results in paralysis of movement of the left eye, with ptosis and dilation of the pupil. An external strabismus is noted, and the eye can be adducted only to the midline. The right side of the body, including the face, shows a loss of tactile, muscle, joint, vibratory, pain, and temperature sense from injury to the ascending sensory tracts; the left medial lemniscus at this level has been joined on its lateral side by the spinothalamic tracts. Involvement of the red nucleus and the superior cerebellar peduncle, which contains efferent fibers from the right cerebellar hemisphere, produces dyssynergia and involuntary movements of the right arm and leg.

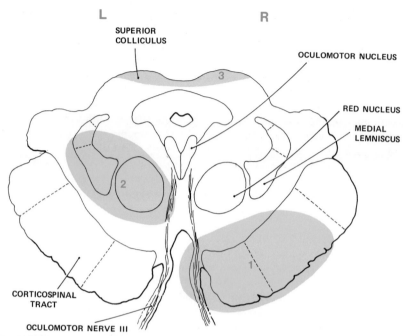

FIGURE 44. A cross section of the midbrain. The shaded areas indicate the positions of lesions. *1.* A lesion of the right cerebral peduncle and oculomotor nerve. Dorsal extension of this lesion will involve the corticobulbar pathway. *2.* A lesion of the tegmentum of the midbrain, affecting the oculomotor nerve, medial lemniscus, red nucleus, and fibers of the superior cerebellar peduncle. *3.* A lesion involving the superior colliculi.

LESIONS OF THE SUPERIOR COLLICULI (PARINAUD'S SYNDROME)

Injury to the superior colliculi (Fig. 44, lesion 3) causes paralysis of upward gaze. The pupils may be fixed or may react in response to accommodation but not to light. This disorder often results from tumors of the pineal gland that compress the superior colliculi.

17

VISION

For vision to occur, reflected rays of light from an object must strike the eye, be refracted by the *cornea* and *lens,* and form an image on the *retina.* The optic principles are the same as those of any camera; the image that is formed is upside-down (inverted) and turned left for right (reversed). The entire visual path within the brain is organized in a fashion that conforms with the peripheral optical system, so that the right hemisphere is presented with upside-down images of objects that lie to the left. This apparent distortion of position, however, is matched by the organization of other systems in the brain. Thus the motor areas of the frontal lobes and the body image contained in the somesthetic zones of the parietal lobe also are inverted and reversed.

THE VISUAL PATHWAY

Light falling on the rods and cones of the retina, the receptors in the visual pathway, triggers a photochemical reaction in these cells. This initiates membrane potential changes in a chain of cells through which nerve impulses are conducted to the cerebral cortex. The first neurons of the visual path are the bipolar cells within the retina. These cells receive input from the receptors and, in turn, synapse with ganglion cells (second-order neurons) of the retina whose axons converge toward the optic disc to form cranial nerve II, the *optic nerve* (Fig. 45). Fibers from the macula, where visual acuity is sharpest, enter the temporal (lateral) side of the optic disc. After perforating the scleral coat of the eye, the optic nerve fibers pass directly to the *optic chiasm,* which is located at the anterior part of the sella turcica of the sphenoid bone immediately in front of the pituitary gland. A partial decussation of fibers takes place in the *chiasm. Fibers from the nasal halves of each retina cross; those from the temporal halves of each retina approach the chiasm and leave it without crossing* (see Fig. 45). Optic fibers continue without any interruption behind the chiasm as two

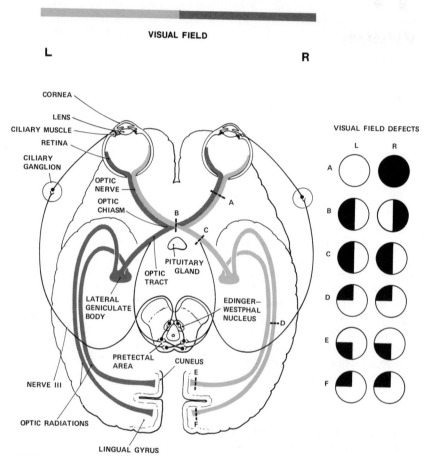

FIGURE 45. The visual pathways. Lesions along the pathway from the eye to the visual cortex *(lesions A through F)* result in deficits in the visual fields, which are shown as black areas on the corresponding visual field diagrams. The pathway through the pretectum and nerve III, which mediates reflex constriction of the pupil in response to light, also is shown.

diverging *optic tracts* that go to the left and right lateral geniculate bodies of the thalamus.

The fibers in front of the chiasm are designated as *optic nerves,* while those behind it are the *optic tracts.* Optic fibers terminate in the *lateral geniculate bodies* (LGB), the *superior colliculus,* and the *pretectal area,* as well as other locations. Cells of the geniculate bodies give rise to fibers that form the *geniculocalcarine tract (optic radiation)* to the cortex of the occipital lobes. The radiation fibers from the lateral part of the LGB are directed downward and forward at first. They then bend backward in a sharp loop and form a flat band that passes through the temporal lobe in the lateral wall of the inferior horn of the lateral ventricle and sweep posteriorly to the occipital lobe. Fibers from the medial portion of the LGB travel adjacent to those from the lateral LGB, but take a more direct, nonlooping course to the occipital lobe. The area of cortex that receives the optic radiations surrounds the *calcarine fissure* on the medial side of the occipital lobe (Fig. 46). The *visual receptive area* (Brodmann's area 17) is also called the striate area because a cross section of the cortex contains a horizontal stripe of white matter within the gray matter (Gennari's line), which is visible to the naked eye. Areas 18 and 19, which adjoin area 17, are important regions for visual perception and for some visual reflexes, such as visual fixation.

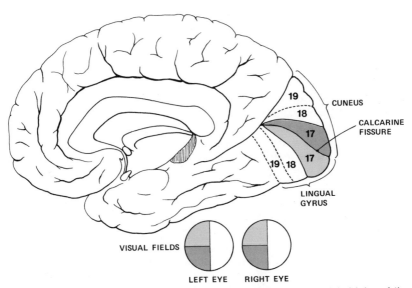

FIGURE 46. The visual cortex on the medial surface of the occipital lobe of the right hemisphere. Note that this brain area receives input from stimuli in the left half of the visual field of each eye.

Effects of Lesions Interrupting the Visual Pathway

Destroying one optic nerve produces blindness in the involved eye (see Fig. 45A). Atrophy of the optic nerves affects some fibers but spares others, and instead of total blindness there usually are areas of lost function in the peripheral part of the fields of vision of each eye. An area of lost function in the visual field is called a *scotoma.*

The *visual fields* can be measured in detail by perimetry, but a simpler way of examining them for gross defects is by the confrontation method. While the subject fixes his gaze straight ahead, the examiner faces the subject and fixes on his eyes. The examiner then introduces an object from some point halfway between himself and the subject but beyond the normal periphery of vision and moves it slowly toward the line of vision. The examiner notes the point at which the object is first seen in his own visual field and by the subject and, after repeating the process in several directions, he makes an estimate of the extent of the field of vision. With optic atrophy both visual fields may be contracted, or a centrally located *scotoma* may be found in each eye. Restricted visual fields, without any organic lesions, are encountered in some psychoneurotic patients to whom everything appears as if viewed through twin gun barrels. These patients, however, do not stumble over objects, and if their visual fields are measured accurately on repeated occasions, gross inconsistencies may be demonstrated.

A lesion of the optic tract behind the chiasm disconnects fibers from one half of each retina. If the right optic tract is destroyed, visual function is lost in the right halves of both retinae. The result, however, is not described in terms of the retinae, but with reference to the disturbance that is produced in the visual fields. In this instance there is blindness for objects in the left half of each field of vision, a condition known as left *homonymous hemianopia* (see Fig. 45C). Even though one optic tract has been completely interrupted, vision sometimes is preserved in a small area at the fixation center, the area of the macula. This phenomenon, called macular sparing, cannot be explained anatomically, and opinions differ as to its significance. Lesions that destroy the entire visual area of the right occipital lobe, or all of the fibers of the right optic radiation, also will produce a left homonymous hemianopia. Visual acuity is not affected in the parts of the retinae whose functions remain, and the patient may not be aware of the presence of a hemianopia.

The *cuneus,* which is the gyrus above the calcarine fissure, receives visual impulses from the dorsal, or upper halves, of the retinae; the *lingual gyrus,* below the calcarine fissure, receives impulses that arise from the ventral, or lower, halves. Thus a lesion that is confined to the right lingual gyrus cuts off visual impulses from the lower part of the right half of each retina. This produces a loss of vision in one quadrant, rather than a hemianopia. Since the images that are focused on the lower part of the retina come from objects above the horizon line, in this instance, an upper left quadrant defect will be found. The visual impulses destined for the lingual gyrus travel in the ventral part of the optic radiation. Consequently, a lesion of the ventral fibers of the right optic radiation has the same effect as a lesion of the right lingual gyrus (see Fig. 45D, E, F).

Lesions of the middle part of the optic chiasm frequently result from compression of these fibers from a tumor of the pituitary gland, or from a craniopharyngioma lying near the midline immediately behind the chiasm. The decussating fibers of the optic nerves are injured, and visual impulses from the nasal halves of each retina are blocked. As a result, the left eye does not perceive images in the left half of its visual field, and the right eye does not record images in the right half of its field of vision. The defect is in the temporal field of each eye and is therefore called *heteronymous bitemporal hemianopia* (see Fig. 45B).

18

OPTIC REFLEXES

THE LIGHT REFLEX

The light reflex consists of the constriction of the pupil that normally occurs when light is flashed into the eye. The sensory receptors for this reflex are the rods and cones of the retina. The afferent pathway follows the course of the visual fibers through the retina, optic nerve and tract as far as the lateral geniculate bodies, but instead of entering the geniculate body, the reflex fibers turn off in the direction of the superior colliculus. They end in a region rostral to the superior colliculus known as the *pretectal area* (see Fig. 45). Interneurons located in this region send axons around the cerebral aqueduct to the *Edinger-Westphal nucleus,* a group of parasympathetic neurons in a rostral subdivision of the oculomotor nuclear complex. The efferent path begins with cells in the Edinger-Westphal nucleus whose axons leave the midbrain in the oculomotor nerve and end in the parasympathetic *ciliary ganglion.* Postganglionic fibers coming from the ganglion enter the eyeball and supply the sphincter muscle in the iris, which constricts the pupil when it contracts.

The response in the eye that has been stimulated by light is termed the *direct reflex.* A *consensual light reflex* is shown by a similar, but weaker, constriction of the pupil of the other eye. The direct light reflex may be abolished by a lesion of the optic nerve or by disease which damages the retina severely. Lesions of the visual path that are located in the lateral geniculate bodies, optic radiations, or visual cortex, however, do not interfere with this reflex. In cortical blindness, produced by a complete destruction of the primary visual areas of both occipital lobes, the light reflexes are preserved. The efferent path for the light reflex may be interrupted by damage to the oculomotor nuclear complex, the oculomotor nerve, or the ciliary ganglion. Neither a direct nor a consensual light reflex then can be obtained on the affected side.

REFLEXES ASSOCIATED WITH THE NEAR-POINT REACTION

When the eyes are directed to an object close at hand, three different reflex responses are brought into cooperative action.

1. *Convergence.* The medial recti muscles contract to move both eyes toward the midline so that the image in each eye remains focused on the fovea (the area of highest acuity within the macula). Without convergence, diplopia, or double vision, occurs.
2. *Accommodation.* The lenses are thickened as a result of tension in the *ciliary muscles* in order to maintain a sharply focused image on the fovea. The ciliary muscles, like the pupillary sphincter, are innervated by postganglionic parasympathetic neurons in the ciliary ganglion.
3. *Pupillary constriction.* The pupils are narrowed as an optical aid to regulate the depth of focus. This constriction does not depend on any change in illumination and is regulated separately from the light reflex.

All three reactions may be initiated by voluntarily directing the gaze to a near object, but an involuntary (reflex) mechanism will accomplish the same results if an object is moved slowly toward the eyes.

THE ARGYLL ROBERTSON PUPIL AND ADIE'S PUPIL

The Argyll Robertson pupil does not react to light but does react to accommodation. The pupil is small and irregular and does not dilate in response to administration of atropine. The Argyll Robertson pupil results from syphilis of the central nervous system, but can occur with other conditions, including diabetes mellitus. The site of the lesion causing the responses of this pupil is unclear, but disease affecting the gray matter about the cerebral aqueduct is likely to be responsible.

Adie's pupil is a benign condition of unknown cause, often seen in young women, consisting of a unilaterally dilated pupil in association with absent deep tendon reflexes. The pupil shows a slow constriction on prolonged exposure to bright light and a more rapid response to accommodation.

THE VISUAL FIXATION REFLEX

Voluntary mechanisms turn the head and eyes toward an object occupying one's attention and bring the desired image into approximately the same position on each retina. The final adjustments, which are necessary to produce identical correspondence of the two visual fields, are carried out by the fixation reflex. If the object is moving, this reflex serves also to hold it in view, involuntarily following its progress by causing appropriate turning movements of both eyes. The afferent pathway of the fixation reflex is from the retina to the visual cortex. The efferent path begins in the cortex of the occipital lobe and goes to the superior colliculus and/or pretectum. Fibers arising from cells in these areas reach the oculomotor nuclei directly and the nuclei of IV and VI indirectly, by way of projections to the paramedian pontine reticular formation and from there to IV and VI via the MLF. When the visual cortex receives images from the left and right retinae that do not match properly, impulses flow through the fibers of the occipitotectal tracts to bring the eyes into correct alignment for fixation.

The fixation reflex is well demonstrated by a passenger viewing the passing scenery from the window of a train. His eyes turn slowly in the direction of apparent movement, then jump ahead quickly to fix the gaze on a new spot. This is done without awareness that the eyes are moving and is called an *optokinetic reflex.*

The fixation reflex is also used during the act of reading. Although we are unaware of it, movement of the eyes along a line of print consists of several jerky movements (saccadic movements) with fixation pauses in between to allow visualization of a group of letters or words. These movements are not under voluntary control. Reading speed can be increased, however, by learning to take in more words at once, or by making the pauses shorter. The difficulty of most slow readers does not lie in the oculomotor reflexes, but in the prolonged time required for each pause.

PROTECTIVE REFLEXES

An object thrust quickly in front of the eyes without warning causes a blink. This reflex response cannot be inhibited voluntarily. Afferent impulses from the retinae go directly to the superior colliculus. From there the impulses are sent in the tectobulbar tracts to the nuclei of the facial nerves and the adjacent reticular formation, which activate the orbicularis oculi muscles and close the lids. A very strong stimulus, such as a sudden blinding flash of light, produces more extensive activity in the tectal region, which sends impulses over tectospinal fibers as well as the tectobulbar tract. Besides closure of the eyes there will be a "startle" response of the whole body musculature, and the arms may be thrown upward across the face. This reflex probably involves tectal input to areas of the reticular formation that project spinalward as well as tectospinal axons.

THE CILIOSPINAL REFLEX

Painful stimulation caused by pinching the skin of the neck or cheek on one side causes dilation of the pupil on the ipsilateral side. This is termed the *ciliospinal reflex.* The afferent limb of the reflex consists of cervical or trigeminal nerves, and the efferent pathway is through the cervical portion of the sympathetic trunk. Postganglionic sympathetic neurons in the superior cervical ganglion send axons which follow the branches of the internal carotid artery to reach the orbit and innervate the dilator muscle of the pupil.

EYE MOVEMENTS

Eye movements are extremely complex and require the integrated function of the cerebral cortex (occipital lobe and frontal eye fields), the cerebellum, the vestibular system, and the reticular formation. All of these systems converge on the oculomotor, trochlear, and abducens nuclei to control the extraocular muscles. Voluntary deviation of the eyes results from the activation of area 8 of Brodmann. The movement of the eyes occurs in the form of *saccades,* which are rapid conjugate movements used to change fixation. Electrical stimulation of area 8 results in conjugate ocular deviation to the opposite side, and damage to this region leads to tonic deviation of the eyes to the ipsilateral side. The pathway for voluntary conjugate ocular deviation involves projections from area 8 of the cerebral cortex through the internal capsule to the ipsilateral superior colliculus. After a synaptic relay, second-order fibers project to the contralateral paramedian pontine reticular formation. Third-order neurons probably connect with neurons in the nuclei of cranial nerves III, IV, and VI.

Reflex slow conjugate movements of the eyes occur without saccades when the eyes follow a moving target. These "pursuit" movements result from activation of areas 17, 18, and 19 in the occipital lobe. The pathway to the nuclei of cranial nerves III, IV, and VI involves synaptic relays in the pretectal and tectal regions. Reflex conjugate ocular movements also can result from vestibular, acoustic, and neck muscle inputs.

19

THE AUTONOMIC NERVOUS SYSTEM

The autonomic nervous system, although a part of the peripheral nervous system, is the functional division that innervates *smooth and cardiac muscle* and the *glands* of the body. By definition it consists of motor *(general visceral efferent)* fibers only; sensory *(general visceral afferent)* fibers accompanying the motor fibers to the viscera are not considered to be a part of the autonomic system. Under ordinary circumstances the autonomic nervous system functions at the subconscious level. It acts to regulate the activity of smooth and cardiac muscles and glands and to integrate these activities with one another and with somatic motor function. However, the organs innervated by the autonomic system can carry out their basic functions (e.g., cardiac contractions, peristalsis of the intestinal tract) without external regulation from the autonomic fibers. In addition to local reflex stimuli, the autonomic neurons are governed by integrative influences from the brain stem and hypothalamus. Unlike the somatic motor system, the autonomic system reaches its effector organs by a two-neuron chain.

The cell bodies and their fibers are classified as follows:

1. The *preganglionic neuron,* the presynaptic or primary neuron, is located in the brain stem (certain cranial nerve nuclei) or spinal cord (intermediolateral gray column).
2. The *postganglionic neuron,* the postsynaptic or secondary neuron, is located in an outlying ganglion and innervates the end organ.

DIVISIONS OF THE AUTONOMIC NERVOUS SYSTEM

The preganglionic fibers have their cell bodies of origin in three regions of the brain stem and spinal cord. The *thoracolumbar outflow* consists of the fibers that arise in the *intermediolateral gray column* of the 12 thoracic and the first two lumbar segments of the spinal cord. This is the *sympathetic division of the autonomic system.* The cranial outflow consists of fibers that arise in the Edinger-Westphal nucleus (cranial nerve III), the superior and inferior salivatory nuclei (cranial nerves VII and IX), and the dorsal motor nucleus of the vagus (cranial nerve X). These fibers follow the cranial nerve branches to their destination. The *sacral outflow* consists of fibers that arise from cell bodies in the intermediate gray matter of *sacral segments 2 through 4.* These fibers form the pelvic splanchnic nerves (nervi erigentes). The cranial and sacral outflow share many anatomic and functional features and together form the *parasympathetic division of the system.*

The sympathetic and parasympathetic divisions of the autonomic nervous system are differentiated not only on their site of origin, but also on the basis of the neurotransmitters released at the terminals of the postganglionic fibers. The terminals of the parasympathetic postganglionic fibers liberate *acetylcholine* and thus are classified as *cholinergic.* The terminals of the sympathetic postganglionic fibers release *norepinephrine* and thus are classified as *adrenergic.* An exception to this rule is found in the terminals of sympathetic fibers on sweat glands, which are cholinergic.

Many organs receive fibers from both the sympathetic and parasympathetic systems. When dual innervation occurs, the fibers frequently have opposing effects. For example, parasympathetic fibers to the stomach increase peristalsis and relax the sphincters, while sympathetic fibers have the opposite effect.

The Sympathetic Nervous System

The myelinated preganglionic fibers (B fibers) of the sympathetic system, which originate in the intermediolateral gray column of the thoracolumbar cord, leave the spinal cord with the motor fibers of the ventral roots but soon separate from the spinal nerves to form the *white rami communicantes* that enter the chain ganglia of the *sympathetic trunks* (see Fig. 9). The trunks are the paired, ganglionated chains of nerve fibers that extend along either side of the vertebral column from the base of the skull to the coccyx. Some of the fibers of the white rami synapse with postganglionic neurons in the trunk ganglion *(paravertebral ganglion)* nearest their point of entrance (see Fig. 9). Other preganglionic fibers pass up or down the chain to end in paravertebral ganglia at higher or lower levels than the point of entrance (not shown in Figure 9). A third group of preganglionic fibers passes through the paravertebral ganglion into a thoracic splanchnic nerve and terminates in the *prevertebral ganglia* of the abdomen and pelvis (see Fig. 9).

Some of the nonmyelinated postganglionic fibers (C fibers) given off from the neurons in the sympathetic trunk ganglia form the gray rami communicantes (see Fig. 9). Each spinal nerve receives a gray ramus that delivers fibers to the spinal cord to be distributed to the blood vessels, erector pili muscles, and sweat glands of the body wall throughout the dermatome innervated by the nerve. There are 31 gray rami on each side of the body, one for each spinal nerve, but there are only 14 white rami. As mentioned above, the white rami carry the preganglionic fibers from the thoracic and upper lumbar segments to the sympathetic chain (trunk). Thus the cervical, lower lumbar, and sacral ganglia of the chain receive preganglionic fibers that have travelled up or down the trunk from the thoracolumbar levels.

The *cervical part* of the sympathetic trunk consists of ascending preganglionic fibers from the first four or five thoracic segments of the spinal cord. Three ganglia are present—*superior cervical, middle cervical,* and *cervicothoracic* (stellate). The last is formed by the fusion of the inferior cervical and first thoracic ganglia. In addition to providing gray rami for the cervical and upper thoracic spinal nerves, the cervical ganglia also give rise to postganglionic fibers in the *cardiac nerves,* which enter the cardiac plexus to supply the sympathetic innervation to the heart. The *carotid plexus* is derived from the superior cervical ganglion. This plexus follows the ramifications of the carotid arteries and furnishes the sympathetic innervation of the head. Some fibers end in blood vessels and sweat glands of the head and face; others supply the lacrimal and salivary glands. The eye receives sympathetic fibers that innervate the dilator muscles of the iris and the smooth muscle fibers of the eyelid.

The viscera of the thorax are supplied not only by the cardiac nerves from the cervical ganglia, but also by postganglionic fibers from the upper thoracic ganglia. These fibers enter the plexuses of the heart and lungs.

The viscera of the abdominal and pelvic cavities are supplied by the thoracic splanchnic nerves. The *thoracic splanchnic nerves* (greater, lesser, and least) carry mainly preganglionic fibers from the spinal cord levels T-5 to T-12, through the sympathetic trunk without synapsing, to the *prevertebral ganglia* of the abdomen. The latter group includes the *celiac, superior mesenteric,* and *aorticorenal* ganglia, which are located at the roots of the arteries for which they are named. The neurons in these ganglia give rise to axons that travel along the arterial walls to reach most of the abdominal viscera. The *lumbar splanchnic nerves* carry the preganglionic fibers from the levels of the upper lumbar spinal cord. The lumbar splanchnics terminate in the *inferior mesenteric* and *hypogastric ganglia.* The postganglionic fibers from these prevertebral (collateral) ganglia follow the ramifications of the visceral arteries to reach the organs of the lower abdomen and pelvis.

Injury to the cervical portion of the sympathetic system produces *Horner's syndrome.* The *pupil* of the injured side is constricted (miotic) because its dilator muscle is paralyzed. There is partial ptosis of the eyelid, but the lid can still be raised voluntarily. An apparent enophthalmos may be noted as well. Absence of *sweating* (anhydrosis) and *vasodilation* on the affected side makes the skin of the face and neck appear reddened, as well as warmer and drier than the normal side. Horner's syndrome may result from lesions that interrupt the central nervous system pathways descending ipsilaterally from the hypothalamus through the brain stem and cervical spinal cord. It can occur when a lesion of the spinal cord destroys the preganglionic neurons at their origin in the upper thoracic segments. Horner's syndrome also follows injury to the cervical sympathetic chain ganglia or the postganglionic fibers.

Sympathetic fibers are known vasoconstrictors, and operations have been devised to increase the circulation by interrupting this innervation. *Lumbar sympathectomy,* which is performed to increase the circulation in the lower extremity, is the most common procedure.

SYMPATHETIC INNERVATION OF THE ADRENAL GLAND

Stimulation of the sympathetic nervous system ordinarily produces generalized physiologic responses rather than discrete localized effects. This results, in part, from the wide dispersion of sympathetic fibers, but it is augmented by the release of epinephrine from the adrenal glands that circulates in the blood. Preganglionic fibers (lesser and least splanchnic nerves) supply the medulla of the adrenal gland, ending directly on the adrenal medullary cells without synapsing in an interposed ganglion. The medullary cells themselves are derivatives of embryonic nerve tissue and, in effect, constitute a modified sympathetic ganglion. Pain, exposure to cold, and strong emotions such as rage and fear evoke sympathetic activity, which mobilizes the body resources for violent action. The functions of the gastrointestinal tract are suspended, and blood is shunted away from the splanchnic area. Heart rate and blood pressure are increased, the coronary arteries dilate, and the bronchioles of the lung widen. The spleen releases extra red cells to the blood. This activity was described by Cannon as the "fight or flight" phenomenon.

The Parasympathetic Nervous System

The preganglionic fibers of the parasympathetic system extend to the *terminal ganglia* located within, or very close to, the organs that they supply. (The myenteric plexus and the ciliary ganglion are respective examples.) The postganglionic fibers, as a result, are very short.

The *cranial division* of the parasympathetic system originates in cranial nerves III, VII, IX, and X. Parasympathetic innervation of the ciliary muscle and sphincter muscle of the iris passes through the oculomotor nerve and ciliary ganglion. Secretory preganglionic fibers from the nervus intermedius of the seventh cranial nerve synapse in the pterygopalatine and submandibular ganglia. Postganglionic fibers from the pterygopalatine ganglion innervate glands in the mucous membrane of the nasal chamber, the air sinuses, the palate and pharynx, and the lacrimal gland, while the fibers of the submandibular ganglion supply the sublingual and submandibular glands. The otic ganglion, which receives preganglionic fibers of the ninth cranial nerve, supplies postganglionic fibers to the parotid gland. The vagus nerve supplies the preganglionic fibers to the heart, lungs, and abdominal viscera. The latter organs have the postganglionic neurons in associated plexuses adjacent to, or within, the walls of the viscus.

The *sacral division* arises from parasympathetic preganglionic neurons in the intermediate gray column of spinal cord segments S-2, S-3, and S-4. Axons of these cells, through the pelvic splanchnic nerves, supply fibers to ganglia in the muscular coats of the urinary and reproductive tracts, the colon (descending and sigmoid), and the rectum. In the pelvic region, the parasympathetic system is primarily concerned with mechanisms for emptying the bladder and rectum. Under strong emotional circumstances these fibers may discharge along with a generalized sympathetic response and produce involuntary emptying of these organs. The parasympathetic fibers are responsible for penile erection, but stimulation by sympathetic fibers initiates the contractions of the ductus deferens and seminal vesicles to produce ejaculation.

INNERVATION OF THE URINARY BLADDER

Motor control of the urinary bladder results primarily from parasympathetic function which, although purely reflex in infants, is under voluntary regulation in normal adults. The preganglionic fibers of the parasympathetic nerves to the bladder have their cell bodies in the intermediate region of the gray matter of sacral cord segments 2, 3, and 4. They enter the pelvic splanchnic nerves, pass through the vesical plexus, and terminate on ganglia located in the wall of the bladder (Fig. 47). Short postganglionic fibers go to the detrusor muscle that forms the wall of the bladder. Stimulation of the parasympathetic nerves of the bladder contracts the detrusor, opens the neck of the bladder into the urethra, and empties the bladder.

The *sympathetic* supply to the bladder originates in cells of the intermediolateral gray column of upper lumbar cord segments whose axons pass through the sympathetic trunk to reach the inferior mesenteric ganglion by the lumbar splanchnic nerves. Postganglionic fibers continue through the hypogastric and vesical plexuses to the wall of the bladder. The functions of the sympathetic nerves are uncertain. They may assist the filling of the bladder by relaxing the detrusor muscle, but they have little influence on emptying mechanisms. Cutting the sympathetic nerves to the bladder does not have a serious effect on its function.

The external sphincter of the urethra is made up of striated muscle and innervated by regular motor fibers of the pudendal nerve along with other muscles of the perineum. The external sphincter may be closed voluntarily but relaxes by reflex action as soon as urine is released into the urethra at the beginning of micturition.

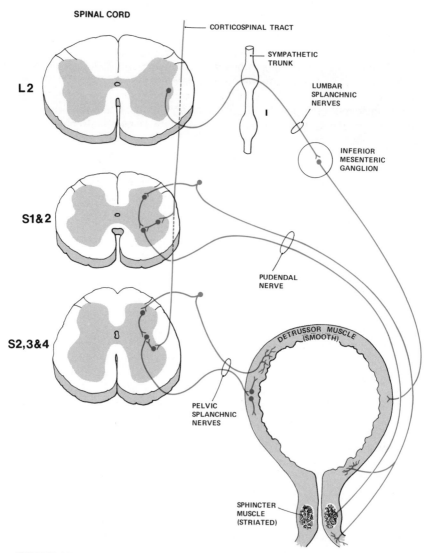

FIGURE 47. Autonomic innervation of the urinary bladder and associated somatic innervation of the sphincter.

The smooth muscle of the bladder responds to a stretch reflex operated by proprioceptors in its wall that send impulses to spinal cord segments S-2, S-3, and S-4. The efferent reflex fibers return impulses over the pelvic splanchnic nerves to maintain tonus in the detrusor muscle while the bladder is filling. In the uninhibited bladder of infancy, the bladder fills nearly to its normal capacity, then a strong reflex response takes place and it empties automatically. Voluntary suppression of urination depends on fibers that descend in the corticospinal tracts from the cortex of the paracentral lobules of the cerebral cortex. These fibers can inhibit the detrusor reflex. The sensation of increased bladder tension and the desire to void are conveyed by sensory impulses in the afferent fibers of the pelvic nerves and visceral afferent pathways deep to the lateral spinothalamic tracts in the lateral funiculus of the spinal cord. The sensations of urethral touch and pressure, however, may be mediated by the dorsal columns.

Lesions of the dorsal roots of the sacral segments interrupt afferent reflex fibers and produce an *atonic bladder*. The bladder wall becomes flaccid and its capacity is greatly increased. Sensations of fullness of the bladder are entirely lost. As the bladder becomes distended, incontinence and dribbling occur. Voluntary emptying remains possible, but it is incomplete and some urine is left in the bladder. Lesions of the conus medullaris of the spinal cord interrupt the central connections of the reflex responsible for emptying the bladder and cause an atonic bladder. Lesions of the cauda equina that destroy the second and third sacral roots interrupt both the afferent and efferent pathways of the reflex and cause an atonic bladder.

Injuries of the spinal cord above the level of the conus medullaris cause a derangement of the bladder reflexes that usually results initially in contraction of sphincter muscles and retention of urine. In the patient with chronic transection of the spinal cord, an *automatic bladder* is frequently established. After several weeks, reflexes in the sacral segments of the cord may recover and begin to function. The bladder fills and empties, either spontaneously or after the skin over the sacral cutaneous area is stimulated by scratching.

20

THE HYPOTHALAMUS AND LIMBIC SYSTEM

THE DIENCEPHALON

The *diencephalon* consists of an ovoid mass of gray matter situated deep in the brain rostral to the midbrain and ventral and caudal to the frontal lobes of the cerebrum. It is separated from the *basal ganglia* by the fibers of the *internal capsule*. Ventrally, it extends from the *optic chiasm* to, and including, the *mammillary bodies*. The rostral limit may be demarcated on a hemisected brain by a line between the *interventricular foramen* and the optic chiasm. The caudal extent is demarcated by a line from the *pineal body* to the mammillary bodies. The third ventricle separates the right half of the diencephalon from the left half, and the roof of this ventricle bears a choroid plexus. In most, but not all, human brains the two halves of the diencephalon are joined at a small area called the *massa intermedia* or *interthalamic adhesion*. Each half of the diencephalon is divided into the following regions: thalamus, hypothalamus, subthalamus, and epithalamus.

The Hypothalamus

The *hypothalamus* forms the floor and the ventral part of the walls of the third ventricle. The shallow *hypothalamic sulcus* on the wall of the third ventricle demarcates the hypothalamus from the thalamus.

The hypothalamus includes a number of well-defined structures. The *optic chiasm* is located at the rostral portion of the hypothalamic floor. The *tuber cinereum* is the portion of the hypothalamic floor between the optic chiasm and the mammillary bodies. The *infundibulum,* or stalk of the pituitary, extends ventrally from the tuber cinereum to the pars nervosa of the hypophysis. The lumen of the third ventricle may evaginate into the infundibulum for a variable distance. The median eminence is a part of the tuber cinereum; it is the portion of the hypothalamic floor between the optic chiasm and the infundibulum. The *mammillary* bodies are paired spherical nuclei located caudal to the tuber cinereum and rostral to the *posterior perforated substance* (Fig. 48).

The hypothalamus consists of three regions: the *supraoptic* region, which is most rostral; the *mammillary* region, which is most caudal; and the intervening *tuberal* region.

HYPOTHALAMIC NUCLEI

The hypothalamus consists of a matrix of nuclei with fiber bundles passing through and between the nuclei. The more conspicuous nuclei in the three major regions are listed below.

Rostral to the hypothalamus is the *preoptic area,* a region developmentally a part of the telencephalon but histologically indistinguishable from the hypothalamus and so closely associated with it functionally that many authorities describe it as part of the hypothalamus. The preoptic area consists of a *medial preoptic area* and a *lateral preoptic area.* The medial preoptic area forms the wall of the third ventricle below the anterior commissure. It extends from the lamina terminalis to an imaginary line running from the interventricular foramen to the back of the optic chiasm (see Fig. 3).

The most rostral portion of the hypothalamus is the supraoptic region, which contains the following structures:

1. The *supraoptic nucleus:* a nucleus that straddles the lateral portions of the optic chiasm.
2. The *paraventricular nucleus:* a group of cells dorsal and medial to the supraoptic nucleus, in the lateral wall of the hypothalamus.
3. The *anterior hypothalamic area:* an indistinctly bounded group of cells between the supraoptic and paraventricular nuclei.
4. The *lateral hypothalamic area:* a long, narrow zone beginning just behind the lateral preoptic area and extending into the intermediate and caudal regions of the hypothalamus. The boundary between the anterior hypothalamic area and the lateral hypothalamic area is a parasagittal plane through the fornix, which is a bundle of fibers traversing the hypothalamus from its dorsorostral corner to the mammillary bodies.

Several small nuclei are found in the tuberal region:

1. The *dorsomedial nucleus,* which is located in the dorsomedial portion of the lateral wall of the ventricle.

2. The *ventromedial nucleus*, which is ventral to the dorsomedial nucleus.
3. The *arcuate nucleus*, which is located in the floor of the hypothalamus near the infundibulum.
4. The *lateral hypothalamic area*, which is lateral to the other three nuclei of this region.

The following nuclei are found in the mammillary region:

1. The *mammillary nuclei*, which are located within the mammillary bodies and usually subdivided into several subnuclei.
2. The *posterior nucleus*, which is dorsal to the mammillary nuclei and caudal to the end of the lateral hypothalamic area.

The preoptic area and hypothalamus are central to the organization of the *limbic system*, which is a collection of interconnected, but not contiguous, structures in the telencephalon. These structures include the cortical areas of the limbic lobe—the cingulate gyrus, septal area, and parahippocampal gyrus (see Chapter 1)—and several gray matter areas beneath the limbic lobe cortex, including the *amygdala* and *hippocampal formation*, which lie deep to the cortex of the parahippocampal gyrus.

The *amygdala* is a spherical mass of neurons that are subdivided into distinct nuclei. These nuclei often are grouped into two functional divi-

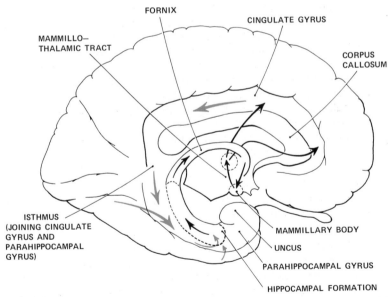

FIGURE 48. The Papez circuit *(arrows)* diagrammed on a schematic view of the limbic system on the medial surface of the cerebral hemisphere.

sions: the dorsomedial and ventrolateral divisions. The amygdala forms the uncus on the parahippocampal gyrus.

Just behind the amygdala is the beginning of the inferior horn of the lateral ventricle, in the floor of which is the *hippocampal formation.* This structure, consisting of the dentate gyrus, Ammon's horn, and the subiculum, is a large gray matter area lying along the ventricle deep to the cortex of the parahippocampal gyrus. It extends from the rostral end of the inferior horn of the lateral ventricle to the back (splenium) of the corpus callosum.

FIBER CONNECTIONS OF THE PREOPTIC AREA AND HYPOTHALAMUS

The preoptic area and hypothalamus receive input from many parts of the limbic system in the telencephalon and from the reticular formation and other nuclei in the brain stem.

Pathways carrying inputs from limbic system structures include the following:

1. The *stria terminalis:* a small, compact bundle of fibers from the dorsomedial division of the amygdala.
2. The *ventral amygdalofugal pathway:* a diffuse projection of axons, probably from both divisions of amygdaloid nuclei, crossing over the optic tract into the hypothalamus and preoptic area.
3. The *fornix:* a large, compact bundle of axons arising from cells of the hippocampal formation. Many fibers in the tract terminate in the mammillary bodies. This tract also includes axons going *to* the hippocampal formation from the hypothalamus and septal area.
4. The *medial forebrain bundle:* a large, somewhat diffuse tract that extends from the septal area through the lateral preoptic area and lateral hypothalamic area to the brain stem, particularly to the reticular formation. Many fibers join this tract and others leave it in all areas through which the tract travels.
5. The *mammillary peduncle:* a pathway carrying fibers from the brain stem into the hypothalamus.

Efferent pathways arising from cells of the hypothalamus travel through the first four tracts listed above. In addition, neurons in the hypothalamus give rise to the following fibers:

1. The *fasciculus mammillary princeps:* a large, short fiber bundle that arises from neurons of the mammillary body, passes dorsally, and bifurcates into the *mammillothalamic tract,* which projects to the anterior nuclear group of the thalamus, and the *mammillotegmental tract,* which turns caudally and terminates in the tegmentum of the midbrain.

2. The *dorsal longitudinal fasciculus:* a small tract connecting the hypothalamus with the brain stem reticular formation and indirectly with cranial nerve nuclei.
3. The *hypothalamo-hypophyseal tract:* fibers from the supraoptic and paraventricular nuclei that send their axons into the posterior lobe of the pituitary.

The functions of the preoptic area and hypothalamus include regulation of (1) body temperature; (2) reproductive physiology and behavior; (3) feeding, drinking, digestion, and metabolic processes of the body, including water balance; and (4) aggressive behavior. In some cases these functions depend upon neurons within the hypothalamus; in other cases these functions result from the actions of pathways such as the medial forebrain bundle that courses through the hypothalamus and connects nonhypothalamic as well as hypothalamic areas. Ambiguities about the functions of local neurons and fibers of passage have resulted in much controversy concerning the functions of the preoptic area and hypothalamus.

In their role as regulator of all the important functions listed above, the preoptic area and hypothalamus are influenced by the major tracts that provide neuronal input as well as by information conveyed to them in the blood stream, such as body core temperature, water and salt content of the blood, and circulating hormone and glucose levels. Similarly, these areas of the brain not only utilize neural effector pathways for their output, but also secrete hormones into the blood stream.

HYPOTHALAMIC PITUITARY RELATIONSHIPS

The hormonal control of the pituitary is mediated, in part, by the direct influence of hormones in the blood on pituitary cells and, in part, by the preoptic area and the supraoptic and tuberal areas of the hypothalamus. These regions influence the anterior and posterior *pituitary* via polypeptides produced in the neurons and transported to their terminals.

Cells in the supraoptic and paraventricular nuclei produce the peptide hormones oxytocin and vasopressin (antidiuretic hormone), which are transported down the *hypothalamo-hypophyseal tract* and secreted from axon terminals directly into the systemic circulation in the posterior pituitary (neurohypophysis).

Cells in the tuberal area control the anterior pituitary, but by a fundamentally different mechanism. Cells in the arcuate nucleus and probably in part of the ventromedial nucleus (as well as cells in more rostral areas of the forebrain) produce *peptide-releasing hormones,* which are transported to their terminals and secreted into capillaries in the median eminence and pituitary stalk. These capillaries collect into very short portal veins that deliver the releasing hormones to cells of the anterior pituitary (adenohypophysis). In response to the appropriate releasing hormones, these cells synthesize and secrete thyroid-stimulating hormone, follicle-stimulating hormone, luteinizing hormone, growth hormone, adrenocorticotropic hormone, and prolactin. These substances are collectively referred to as trophic hormones because they have a stimulating effect on their target tissues. In response many of the target tissues (e.g., thyroid and adrenal glands) produce hormones that serve as negative feedback regulators on the hypothalamus and pituitary. This is not true of the regulation of growth hormone and prolactin, which are controlled by a balance of stimulating and inhibiting "releasing hormones" from the hypothalamus.

BODY TEMPERATURE

The preoptic area and the anterior hypothalamic area are important in temperature regulation. Damage to these areas of the brain can lead to complete loss of the integration of autonomic reflexes (e.g., peripheral vasoconstriction or vasodilatation and sweating) and somatic motor or behavioral responses (e.g., shivering and moving to a warmer or cooler environment) that regulate body temperature. In addition, local cooling or warming of the blood supply in this area produces an appropriate set of compensatory responses to maintain body temperature at 37°C. Neurons in the preoptic and hypothalamic regions appear to be directly responsible for this regulatory function. These neurons probably control the production of fever as well, but the mechanisms involved are not fully understood.

REPRODUCTIVE PHYSIOLOGY AND BEHAVIOR

Neurons in the preoptic area, anterior hypothalamus, and tuberal region are involved in gonadal regulation and sexual behavior in the male and female. Both anatomic and physiologic differentiation of these brain areas occurs in response to gonadal hormones circulating before birth, leading to a postpubertal pattern of cyclical (female) or noncyclical (male) secretion of gonadotropin-releasing hormone (GnRH). Neurons in the arcuate nucleus, in part of the ventromedial nucleus in the tuberal region, and probably also in the preoptic region are directly responsible for synthesizing GnRH, transporting it down their axons, and secreting it into the portal capillaries in the infundibulum. Neurons in these same areas influence sexual behavior profoundly in all experimental animals in which this question has been studied, but the pathways out of the hypothalamus by which sexual behavior is coordinated are not fully known. Certainly, some of this behavioral integration involves hypothalamic output to the parasympathetic and sympathetic preganglionic neurons that control genital reflexes.

The neuronal inputs to the preoptic area and hypothalamus that influence sexual behavior come from the amygdala and the brain stem. In addition, the blood-borne gonadal hormones, estrogen and progesterone or testosterone, are accumulated by neurons in the medial preoptic area and tuberal hypothalamus. These hormones may influence the electrical activity of the neurons in addition to controlling the synthesis and release of GnRH.

FOOD INTAKE

Damage to the ventromedial nucleus of the hypothalamus causes an experimental animal to eat voraciously. If allowed continuous access to food, such an animal quickly becomes obese. Conversely, a lesion placed in the lateral hypothalamic area in the tuberal region abolishes eating and drinking behavior, at least temporarily, and may lead to death from loss of water and nourishment. These experimental findings led investigators to designate the neurons of the ventromedial nucleus "the satiety center" and those of the lateral hypothalamic area "the feeding center." Further experiments have suggested that pathways passing through these areas may be as important as the neurons located there. The neuronal mechanisms controlling feeding and drinking behaviors are still being investigated. Undoubtedly they involve the function of a number of brain areas outside the hypothalamus as well as the tuberal neurons.

EMOTION

The hypothalamus clearly regulates the autonomic discharge of nerve impulses that evoke the physical expressions of emotion: acceleration of the heart rate, elevation of blood pressure, flushing (or pallor) of the skin, sweating, "goose-pimpling" of the skin, dryness of the mouth, and disturbances of the gastrointestinal tract. However, emotional experience includes subjective aspects or "feelings" that are likely to involve the cerebral cortex. Furthermore, mental processes in the cerebral cortex possessing strong emotional content can bring forth hypothalamic reactions. Pathways that connect the cerebral cortex and hypothalamus therefore are intimately involved in the mechanisms of emotion.

Conduction pathways between the hypothalamus and the cerebral cortex are diverse and circuitous. One of the most direct is a pathway known as the Papez circuit. Papez's description of this pathway and his proposal that it is concerned with emotion led the way in the development of the concept of the limbic system. The pathway includes the hippocampal formation, a primitive cortical area that receives substantial input from the association cortex in the parahippocampal gyrus. The hippocampal formation projects directly to the hypothalamus, particularly the mammillary body, via the fornix. From the mammillary body the prominent mammillothalamic tract projects to the anterior nuclear group of the thalamus, and from these nuclei axons distribute to the cingulate gyrus.

Ironically, although the limbic system as a whole has been shown to be concerned with emotion, as Papez proposed for the hippocampus, the hippocampus itself has been studied most extensively as an area of the brain responsible for laying down memories—an area, therefore, of prime importance in learning.

21

THE THALAMUS

The thalamus comprises the dorsal portion of the diencephalon. The relation to the hypothalamus and subthalamus has been described previously. The thalamus is bounded medially by the wall of the third ventricle and laterally by the posterior limb of the internal capsule. The dorsal surface of the thalamus has been covered by the overgrowth of the forebrain. A groove, the *terminal sulcus,* which contains the *stria terminalis* and terminal vein, demarcates the thalamus from the caudate nucleus along the dorsolateral margin of the thalamus.

The thalamus is subdivided into three unequal parts by the *internal medullary lamina.* This band of myelinated fibers demarcates the medial and lateral nuclear masses (Fig. 49B), and bifurcates at its rostral extent to encompass the anterior nucleus. The centromedian nucleus and other intralaminar nuclei are enclosed within the internal medullary lamina in the center of the thalamus.

The thalamus serves as the station from which, after synaptic interruption and processing, impulses of all types are relayed to the cerebral cortex. It is an important general principle that thalamic nuclei projecting to a specific region of the cerebral cortex also receive afferents (corticothalamic fibers) from that same cortical region. Correlation and integration of information occur within the thalamus, but conscious interpretation of peripheral sensory stimuli, except for pain, does not occur at this level. The thalamus may be concerned with the focusing of attention, perhaps by temporarily making certain cortical sensory areas especially receptive and others less receptive.

THALAMIC NUCLEI AND THEIR CONNECTIONS

Medial Nuclear Mass

The *medial nuclear mass* (located medial to the internal medullary lamina) contains one major nucleus, the *dorsomedial nucleus* (DM) (Fig. 49A, B), which is subdivided into *small cell (parvocellular)* and *large cell (magnocellular)* components. The small cell portion has a reciprocal relationship with most of the prefrontal cortex of the frontal lobe (Fig. 49C, D), which is involved in affective aspects of sensory experience. The large cell component is interrelated with the hypothalamus, the amygdala, and the orbital portion of the frontal lobe and may be involved in olfactory discrimination as well as other, as yet undefined functions. The DM nucleus has many interconnections with other thalamic nuclei, including the intralaminar and midline nuclei and the lateral thalamic nuclear mass.

Midline Nuclei

Midline nuclei are very diffuse, small nuclei located in the periventricular region and in the interthalamic adhesion. They are interconnected with structures in the basal forebrain and limbic system.

Lateral Nuclear Mass

The *lateral nuclear mass* (located lateral to the internal medullary lamina) is subdivided into a dorsal and a ventral tier of nuclei (Fig. 49A).

The *dorsal tier of nuclei* includes, in a rostrocaudal direction:

1. The *lateral dorsal nucleus* (LD), which can be considered as the caudal extension of the anterior thalamic nucleus (A), and which interconnects with the cingulate gyrus and precuneus.
2. The *lateral posterior nucleus* (LP), which is reciprocally connected with the caudal aspect of precuneus and with the superior parietal lobule (areas 5 and 7). It receives input from the superior colliculus and other thalamic nuclei.
3. The *pulvinar nucleus* (P), which is a large nucleus in the posterolateral portion of the thalamus. It connects reciprocally with large association areas of the parietal, temporal, and occipital lobes of the cerebral cortex. Similar to the LP nucleus, it receives input from the superior colliculus, retina, cerebellum, and other thalamic nuclei.

The *ventral tier of nuclei* includes, in a rostrocaudal direction:

1. The *ventral anterior nucleus* (VA), which is subdivided into *small* and *large cell* populations. The large cell component receives its

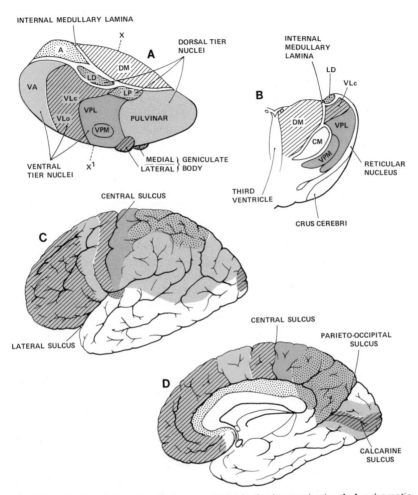

FIGURE 49. The thalamocortical connections in the human brain. *A.* A schematic dorsolateral view of the thalamus, which has been dissected from the left side of the brain, showing the boundaries of the major nuclei. (A = anterior nuclear group; DM = dorsomedial nucleus; LD = lateral dorsal nucleus; LP = lateral posterior nucleus; VA = ventral anterior nucleus; VLC = ventral lateral pars caudalis; VLO = ventral lateral pars oralis; VPL = ventral posterolateral; VPM = ventral posteromedial nucleus.) The reticular nucleus is omitted to expose the ventral tier nuclei. *B.* A coronal section through the thalamus and subthalamus, showing the plane of a section through XX'. Also shown is the centromedian (CM), which is one of the intralaminar nuclei. *C.* The lateral surface of the cerebral cortex. Shaded and colored areas on the cortex designate the correspondingly shaded thalamic nuclei with which these cortical areas are interconnected. *D.* The medial surface of the cerebral cortex.

input from the substantia nigra (SN), and the small cell portion receives fibers from the medial aspect of the globus pallidus (GP). The VA nucleus also receives fibers from other thalamic nuclei (intralaminar and midline), the brain stem reticular formation, and the cerebral cortex. It projects to the frontal lobe, particularly to area 6 in the premotor cortex, including the *supplementary motor cortex* located on the medial aspect of the superior frontal gyrus immediately rostral to area 4 (see Figs. 50 and 51).

2. The *ventral lateral nucleus* (VL), which is similar to the VA nucleus in that it contains both *small and large cell components* that receive fibers from the GP and SN respectively. It also receives fibers from other thalamic nuclei, the brain stem reticular formation, and the cerebral cortex. It may differ from the VA nucleus in that it receives a major input from the cerebellum. Contrary to earlier ideas, it appears not to receive input from the red nucleus. It is reciprocally connected to the *precentral gyrus* (area 4), which is the *primary motor region* of the cerebral cortex.

3. The *ventral posterior nuclear complex* (VP), which is referred to as the ventrobasal complex by physiologists, and consists of two major subdivisions: the *ventral posteromedial nucleus* (VPM), which is also called the semilunar or arcuate nucleus, and the *ventral posterolateral nucleus* (VPL). Some authorities include a third, smaller component, the ventral posterointermediate nucleus (VPI), which is sandwiched in between the VPL and VPM nuclei. The VP nuclear complex is the main somatosensory and taste region of the thalamus. Many of the cells in this complex are both place- and modality-specific and have small receptive fields. It is a synaptic station for the medial lemniscus, the gustatory pathways, the secondary trigeminal tracts, and part of the spinothalamic system. The sensory tracts from the head, including the gustatory pathways, terminate in the VPM nucleus, while those from the remainder of the body synapse in the VPL nucleus. Consequently, the VP nuclear complex is *somatotopically organized* such that the input from the lower portion of the body is most laterally represented and that from the upper part most medially. This nuclear complex projects primarily to the *postcentral gyrus* areas 3, 2, and 1, the *primary somesthetic cortex.* The postcentral gyrus is somatotopically organized such that the face is represented ventrolaterally (thus receiving the projection from VPM), and the leg dorsomedially (receiving its input from the VPL). The VP nuclear complex also projects to the *secondary somesthetic cortex,* which is located in the most ventral aspect of the precentral gyrus (the superior lip of the lateral cerebral fissure) and extends caudally to some extent in the parietal lobe.

4. The *posterior nuclear group (PO),* which is a region of the thalamus located just caudal to the VP complex, medial to the medial geniculate body (MG), and ventral to the pulvinar nucleus (P). It receives a

bilateral input from the spinal cord and is not somatotopically organized. Its neurons have large, diffuse receptive fields. Other sensory
modalities also project to this nucleus. The PO complex projects
primarily to the *secondary somesthetic cortex.*

5. The *metathalamic nuclei,* which include the medial (MG) and lateral
   (LG) geniculate bodies:
   a. The *medial geniculate body* (MG) lies adjacent to the superior
      colliculus and receives bilateral auditory impulses from the nu-
      cleus of the inferior colliculus (IC) and some fibers from more
      caudal auditory nuclei through the brachium of the IC. The MG
      projects, through the auditory radiations, to the auditory cortex
      of the superior temporal gyrus, specifically to the transverse gy-
      rus of Heschl, area 41 (see Figs. 49C and 50).
   b. The *lateral geniculate body* (LG) is the main portion of this nu-
      clear complex in primates and contains six layers of cells. It
      receives fibers from both eyes, but the optic tract fibers originat-
      ing in the left eye distribute to only three of the six layers, and
      those from the right eye distribute to the remaining three layers.
      Thus there are no lateral geniculate cells with binocular recep-
      tive fields. The LG is *reciprocally connected* via the optic radi-
      ations (the geniculocalcarine tract) to the visual cortex of the
      occipital lobe, area 17, which is on the medial surface of the
      hemisphere (see Figs. 49D and 51). In the visual cortex, many of
      the cells have binocular receptive fields (i.e., they can be excited
      by light from an object when it falls on the appropriate receptive
      field area of either eye). This is because LG cells from the same
      part of the LG, but from alternate layers of cells, converge on
      individual occipital cortex neurons. The LG also is intercon-
      nected with the pulvinar and other thalamic nuclei.

Anterior Nucleus

The *anterior nucleus* (A) is actually a complex of three nuclei located in the
conspicuous anterior tubercle of the thalamus. This nucleus, in which the
mammillothalamic tract and fibers from the hippocampus terminate, has
reciprocal connections with the cingulate gyrus and the hypothalamus.
This is an important relay nucleus in the *limbic system.*

Intralaminar Nuclei

Intralaminar nuclei are numerous small, diffuse collections of nerve cells
within the internal medullary lamina. In the caudal aspect of the lamina
there are two more circumscribed intralaminar nuclei that can be delin-
eated: the *centromedian nucleus (CM),* which lies adjacent to the VP complex, and the *parafascicular nucleus* (PF), which is located immediately
medial to the CM nucleus.

In general, the intralaminar nuclei represent the rostral extent of the ascending *reticular system*. They are interconnected with other thalamic nuclei and receive bilateral input from the anterolateral system. The CM nucleus receives fibers from the globus pallidus (GP) and area 4 of the cerebrum and, in conjunction with the PF nucleus, projects to the putamen and caudate nucleus. The PF nucleus receives fibers from area 6 of the cerebrum. Axon collaterals of the fibers to the putamen and caudate nucleus project onto the cerebral cortex.

Thalamic Reticular Nucleus

The *thalamic reticular nucleus* is a thin layer of cells sandwiched between the posterior limb of the internal capsule and the external medullary lamina. It is actually a derivative of the ventral thalamus. There is disagreement as to whether this nucleus should be considered part of the reticular system. It does not project fibers to the cerebral cortex; instead it sends fibers to the thalamic nuclei, the brain stem reticular formation, and other parts of the thalamic reticular nucleus. It does receive fibers from the cerebrum. Nearly all thalamic efferent fibers to the cortex must pass through this nuclear complex. In doing so, they may send collaterals to the cells in the area. Consequently, the reticular nucleus may be important in the regulation of thalamic activity, though its function has not been defined. The feedback of the cerebral cortex to this nucleus may provide a mechanism with which the cerebrum can screen the information that it receives.

FUNCTIONAL CATEGORIZATION OF THALAMIC NUCLEI

Functionally, the thalamic nuclei have been categorized as either specific or nonspecific. This nomenclature was based on the electrophysiologic responses evoked in the cerebral cortex after stimulation of individual thalamic nuclei. "Nonspecific" nuclei were those that produced evoked potentials over large areas of the cortex, in contrast to localized responses following stimulation of "specific" nuclei.

Anatomic nomenclature for groups of thalamic nuclei is based on similarities in their patterns of connections. In this system, three groups are frequently identified:

1. *Specific nuclei* have reciprocal relations with specific areas of the cerebrum known to have specific sensory or motor functions. They receive an input from the ascending pathways or major relay nuclei and include most of the ventral tier nuclei of the lateral nuclear mass: the LG, MG, VA (in part), VL, and VP nuclei.
2. *Association nuclei* do not receive direct input from ascending tracts. They have reciprocal connections with the association areas of the

cerebral cortex. The main structures included are the dorsal tier nuclei in the lateral nuclear mass: the LD, LP, and pulvinar nuclei. The parvocellular component of the DM nucleus and the anterior nuclei also are included.

3. *Subcortical nuclei* have no direct afferent or efferent connections with the cerebral cortex and include the DM (in part), VA (in part), intralaminar, and thalamic reticular nuclei.

THE EPITHALAMUS

The epithalamus is the most dorsal division of the diencephalon. The major structures of this region are the pineal body (epiphysis), the habenular nuclei and commissure, the posterior commissure, the striae medullares, and the roof of the third ventricle.

The *pineal body* is the dorsal diverticulum of the diencephalon. It is a cone-shaped structure that overlies the tectum of the midbrain. Microscopically, it consists of glial cells (astrocytes) and parenchymal cells (pinealocytes). No neurons are present, but there is an abundance of nerve fibers serving primarily as the terminals of postganglionic sympathetic neurons in the superior cervical ganglion. Calcareous accumulations (corpora arenacea) are conspicuous features of the pineal body after middle age. Since the pineal body is normally a midline structure and its calcifications often are radiopaque, its position can be a useful diagnostic aid on routine skull films. The function of the pineal has been a controversial subject. In many vertebrates the secretions of the pinealocytes (including melatonin) are involved in seasonal maintenance and regression of gonadal cycling. The function of the pineal in the human is not known.

The *habenular nuclei* are located in the dorsal margin of the base of the pineal body. Afferent fibers to the habenula originate in the septal area, the lateral hypothalamus, and the brain stem, including the interpeduncular nucleus, the raphe nuclei, and the ventral tegmental area. These brain stem afferents reach the habenula in the *habenulopeduncular tract,* while the more rostral afferents are carried in the *stria medullaris.* The stria medullaris forms a small ridge on the dorsomedial margin of the thalamus. The efferent fibers of the habenula in the *habenulopeduncular tract,* or fasciculus retroflexus, are contained in a conspicuous, dense bundle that terminates in the interpeduncular nucleus. Fibers from the latter nucleus include ascending projections to the thalamus, hypothalamus, and septal area and descending fibers that terminate in the central gray matter and serotonergic raphe nuclei of the brain stem.

The *habenular commissure* consists of stria medullaris fibers crossing over to the contralateral habenular nuclei. The *posterior commissure,* located ventral to the base of the pineal body, carries decussating fibers of the superior colliculi and pretectum (visual reflex fibers), and possibly fibers from other sources.

22

THE RHINENCEPHALON
AND OLFACTORY REFLEXES

The rhinencephalon consists of the olfactory nerves, bulbs, tracts and striae, a portion of the anterior perforated substance, the prepyriform region of the cortex, the entorhinal cortex of the parahippocampal gyrus, and the corticomedial (dorsomedial) division of the amygdala. The rhinencephalon is relatively prominent in the brain of macrosmatic vertebrates such as carnivores and rodents. In microsmatic vertebrates such as primates, the visual sense is used more extensively than the olfactory for locating food and for communication with other members of the same species.

PERIPHERAL OLFACTORY APPARATUS

The peripheral olfactory receptors are found in a specialized area of the nasal mucosa designated as the *olfactory epithelium.* In humans, this pseudostratified columnar olfactory epithelium is located on the superior concha, the roof of the nasal chamber, and the upper portion of the nasal septum. The receptor cells are bipolar neurons. Their axons, grouped into fascicles, pass through the fenestra of the cribriform plate as the olfactory nerve. The olfactory nerves terminate in the *olfactory bulb,* which is an extension of the telencephalon.

OLFACTORY BULBS AND OLFACTORY STRIAE

The olfactory bulbs rest on the cribriform plate. The laminar architecture of the bulb is prominent in histological preparations of most vertebrate brains but difficult to demonstrate in humans. The bulb contains several types of neurons, including interneurons and mitral cells, which receive input from olfactory *nerve fibers* and project their axons into the olfactory tracts or striae.

The *anterior olfactory nucleus,* in the olfactory stalk, consists of a number of groups of neurons. It contains the cells of origin of the olfactory portion of the anterior commissure. These cells receive input from the olfactory bulb rostrally and send their axons across the anterior commissure to the contralateral olfactory bulb.

The olfactory stalk lies in the olfactory sulcus. The tract in the stalk soon bifurcates into medial and lateral striae. Some of the fibers of the medial olfactory stria are the axons of anterior olfactory nucleus neurons, which enter the rostral portion of the anterior commissure to be returned to the opposite olfactory bulb. The remainder of the fibers, which terminate in the olfactory trigone within the anterior perforated substance, are believed to be mitral cell axons.

The lateral stria, composed primarily of mitral cell processes, skirts the lateral margin of the anterior perforated substance to reach the prepyriform cortex, the entorhinal cortex, and the amygdala. The olfactory system is unusual in that it is the only sensory system in which second-order neurons project directly to the cortex. The primary olfactory cortex (prepyriform cortex) is three-layered paleocortex, which is phylogenetically older than the six-layered neocortex in which visual, auditory, and somatosensory systems terminate. However, the olfactory system, like these other sensory systems, does use a thalamocortical connection to the *neocortex* for discriminative functions. This connection includes projections from the primary olfactory cortex to the dorsomedial nucleus of the thalamus, which relays information to the orbitofrontal cortex. Experimental animals in which this system has been damaged can still respond to the presence of an odor, but they cannot discriminate one odorant from another.

Olfactory impulses that reach the amygdala are involved in regulation of chemosensory control of social behaviors in macrosmatic vertebrates. These behaviors include sexual, aggressive, and maternal responses to other members of the same species. The functional significance of olfactory projections to the amygdala in primates is not clear, nor is the function of the olfactory input to the entorhinal cortex. It is likely that in both of these regions, olfactory information is integrated with visual, auditory, and somatosensory impulses arriving from their respective association cortices. The entorhinal area projects heavily to the hippocampal formation. Thus both the amygdala and the hippocampal formation may be involved in the integration of multisensory inputs into meaningful and appropriate emotional and physiologic responses to external stimuli. This would serve as the groundwork for development of learned emotional responses to specific stimuli, an aspect of motivation.

Anosmia, a loss of the sense of smell, can result from a number of conditions, including trauma (fracture of the cribriform plate with injury to the olfactory bulbs or tracts); infections (the common cold and other systemic viral infections such as viral hepatitis, syphilis, bacterial meningitis, abscesses of the frontal lobe, and osteomyelitis of the frontal or ethmoid regions); neoplasms (olfactory groove meningiomas and frontal lobe gliomas); metabolic diseases (pernicious anemia and disorders of zinc metabolism); and drug ingestion (especially of amphetamine and cocaine). Hyperosmia, an increase in olfactory sensitivity, occurs most frequently in hysteria and some psychoses.

The subarachnoid space is located in close approximation to the olfactory mucosa. A fracture through the cribriform plate can result in a leak of cerebrospinal fluid through the nose (CSF rhinorrhea). This condition can result in meningitis due to the spread of infection from the nose to the cerebrospinal fluid.

23

THE CEREBRAL CORTEX

The advanced intellectual functions of the human depend upon the activity of the cerebral cortex and interactions of this structure with other portions of the nervous system. The cerebral cortex is involved in many aspects of memory storage and recall. It is necessary for the comprehension and execution of language and for certain special talents such as musical and mathematical abilities. The cerebral cortex is involved in most higher cognitive functions. It is responsible for the perception and conscious understanding of many sensations applied to the body surface, as well as hearing and vision. It is an important site in which one modality of sensation can be integrated with others, and in which ongoing sensations can be related to past experiences. The cerebral cortex is involved in the processing of many complex motor activities, particularly fine digital and hand movements.

NEURONS OF THE CEREBRAL CORTEX

The convoluted surface of the cerebral hemispheres contains a mantle of gray matter, thickly studded with cells that are arranged in layers. The *iso-cortex* (neocortex), which comprises about 90 percent of the cerebral surface, contains six layers of cells, while the *allocortex* contains three. The allocortex includes the *paleocortex* (e.g., olfactory cortex), and the *archi-cortex* (e.g., hippocampus and dentate gyrus). A third region of the cerebral surface, including the cingulate gyrus and part of the parahippocampal gyrus, is transitional from allocortex to isocortex and contains between three and six neuronal layers, depending upon the location. From the pial surface, the layers of the neocortex have been named: I, *molecular;* II, *external granular;* III, *external pyramidal;* IV, *internal granular;* V, *internal pyramidal;* and VI, *multiform.* In general, afferents to the cortex synapse in layers I through IV, while efferents leaving the cortex arise from layers V and VI. In addition to this horizontal lamination, the cells of the cortex are functionally organized into vertical columns. Afferent fibers to the cortex run radially toward the surface (i.e., along the length of the vertical columns) or in sheets between the layers of cells. The vertical columns are extremely important and are considered to be the functional units of the cortex. Short axons make connections between neurons within each column to form a great variety of closed chains, or loops. Some of the fibers which terminate on the cells of the cortex come from the thalamus *(projection fibers)* primarily to layer IV; others arrive from widely dispersed areas of the cortex by way of long or short *association fibers.* A third group of fibers projects to the cortex from several specific subcortical structures outside the thalamus. These include the locus ceruleus (origin of noradrenergic fibers), the raphe nuclei of the brain stem (origin of serotonin projections), and the basal nucleus of Meynert (in the basal telencephalon; origin of acetylcholine projections). The corpus callosum *(commissural fibers)* links corresponding (and to some degree, noncorresponding) regions of the two hemispheres.

The relative thickness of each of the six cortical layers, and the density of neuron cell bodies within each layer, varies in different regions of the cortex. On the basis of such morphologic characteristics—some obvious, others very subtle—several cytoarchitectural maps have been developed, dividing the surface of the cerebrum into distinct areas. Some areas have recognized functions, but for many no clear correspondence with a specific function has been proved. Based on the differences in cytoarchitecture, Brodmann designated 52 anatomic areas. Several of these are used frequently for descriptive purposes (Figs. 50 and 51).

Motor Functions of the Cerebral Cortex

The *primary motor region* (area 4) is located in the precentral gyrus on the convexity of the cerebral hemisphere, extending from the Sylvian fissure laterally into the interhemispheric fissure medially. The largest neuronal cell bodies of the cerebral cortex, the Betz cells, are located in layer V of this region. They give rise to a very small percentage of the fibers in the corticospinal tract. The other, smaller neurons in area 4 give rise to a significant portion of the corticospinal tract. As shown by the effects of electrical stimulation in humans and animals, this area of the cerebral cortex contains a representation of the muscles of the body in an orderly arrangement (Fig. 52). The toes, ankle, leg, and genitalia are represented on the medial

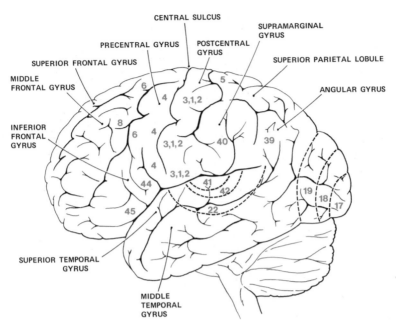

FIGURE 50. A lateral view of the surface of the brain, showing some of the important areas of Brodmann.

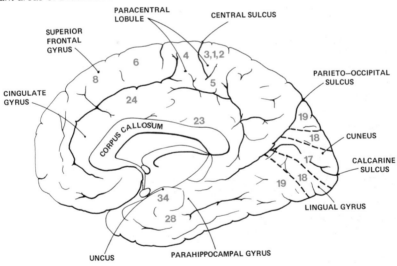

FIGURE 51. A medial view of the surface of the brain, showing some of the important areas of Brodmann.

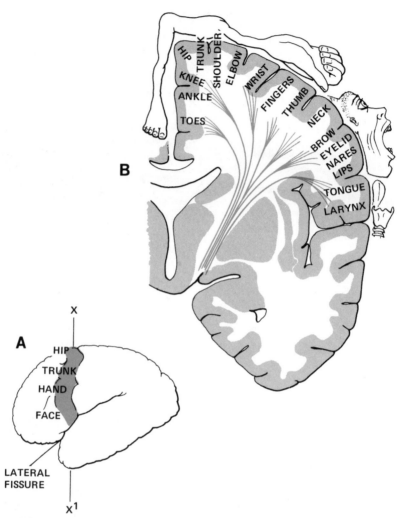

FIGURE 52. A cross section through the precentral region of the cerebral hemisphere, as shown in the inset *(A)*. The section *(B)*, which was taken at coronal plane XX', shows the topographic representation of the opposite side of the body in the motor area of the left frontal lobe. (Modified from Penfield, W., and Rasmussen, H.: *The Cerebral Cortex in Man.* Macmillan, New York, 1950.)

wall of the brain, and the knee, hip, and trunk follow in sequence on the convexity. The shoulder, elbow, wrist, and fingers occur next, and the neck, brow, face, lips, jaw, and tongue are represented most laterally. The amounts of cortex devoted to various parts of the body are unequal. The parts of the body capable of fine or delicate movement have a large cortical representation, whereas those performing relatively gross movements have a smaller representation.

Lesions in the primary motor region result in paresis of the contralateral musculature with hypotonia (decreased resistance to passive manipulation) and diminished muscle stretch reflexes. This is followed in a few weeks by spasticity of the affected musculature with hypertonia (increased resistance to passive manipulation), enhanced muscle stretch reflexes, and an extensor plantar response (Babinski sign).

A *supplementary motor area* is present on the medial surface of the cerebral hemisphere, in area 6, just rostral to the primary motor area (Fig. 53). This area contains a complete somatotopic representation of the body. A third motor representation exists in the postcentral region of the cerebral cortex. The body components of this representation coincide with the somatic sensory pattern in the same area. All four of the areas of cerebral

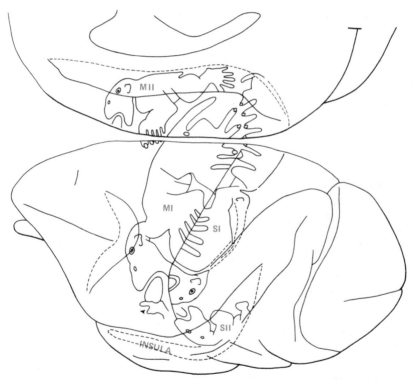

FIGURE 53. Diagram of the cerebral cortex of the monkey, showing the locations of four principal motor areas: precentral motor, MI; supplementary motor, MII; somatic sensory I, SI; and secondary sensory, SII. The figurines in the diagram indicate the segments of the body induced to move by electrical stimulation. (Modified from Harlow, H. F., and Woolsey, C. N. (eds.): *Biological and Biochemical Bases of Behavior.* University of Wisconsin Press, Madison, 1958.)

cortex containing motor representation send fibers into the pyramidal tract, and all probably provide inputs to motor pathways other than the pyramidal as well.

The motor cortex is organized in a columnar arrangement with radially arranged columns of neurons extending vertically from the surface into the depths of the cortex. A single column is a functional entity responsible for directing a group of muscles acting on a single joint. With this organization, movements, and not individual muscles, are represented in the motor cortex. Individual muscles are represented repeatedly, in different combinations, among the columns.

The premotor area (area 6) lies immediately in front of area 4, and continues on the medial surface to the cingulate gyrus. Area 6 contains neurons providing inputs both to the pyramidal tract and to extrapyramidal pathways. Area 8 lies rostral to area 6, and contains the frontal eye field. Stimulation of this area results in conjugate deviation of the eyes to the opposite side. This region is responsible for voluntary conjugate movement of the eyes, independent of visual stimuli. Another motor eye field is located in a large region of the occipital lobe, including the visual receiving areas and adjacent zones of the cerebral cortex. The site of lowest threshold for a response to electrical stimulation is area 17. This area subserves movements of the eyes induced by visual stimuli, as in following moving objects.

Prefrontal Cortex

The large remaining part of the frontal lobe lying rostral to the motor and premotor areas is known as the *prefrontal region* and includes areas 9 through 12. Besides its connections with the dorsomedial nucleus of the thalamus, this part of the cerebral cortex receives connections from the anterior portions of the temporal lobe and from the parietal and occipitotemporal association areas. It is believed that this region is essential for abstract thinking, foresight, mature judgment, tactfulness, and forebearance. These regions do not, however, seem to be primarily concerned with intelligence as it is customarily tested.

The *symptoms* of patients with disease of the prefrontal cortex, as, for example, in patients with brain tumors of this area, are chiefly mental. A diminished sense of responsibility in personal affairs may be noted, as well as slovenliness in personal habits, vulgarity in speech, and clownish behavior, frequently accompanied by feelings of euphoria. The patient lacks judgment, insight, and concern for the future effects of immediate decisions.

The operation of *prefrontal leukotomy* (or *lobotomy*) consists of severing the connections of the prefrontal area with the dorsomedial nucleus of the thalamus by passing a cutting instrument through the roof of the orbit and sweeping it across the fibers in a coronal plane. Identical effects have been produced by passing a needle into the dorsomedial nucleus and destroying it by cautery. At one time these operations were used extensively in attempts to rehabilitate psychotic patients and to relieve patients with chronic intractable pain of organic origin. The results in psychotic patients permitted many to return home from institutions and some to be gainfully employed. Patients operated upon for pain no longer complained of pain or appeared to be in distress, although they stated that pain was still present. Relief was due to loss of the fear and anxiety that were associated with the pain. These results were achieved with many undesirable side effects. The patients were careless with personal habits, unaffected by criticism, unconcerned with social relationships, tactless, and easily amused. They were oblivious to financial and domestic difficulties and could not appreciate the gravity of situations or maintain a responsible attitude toward them. In current practice, prefrontal leukotomy is performed only rarely, since advances in drug therapy have made it possible to treat psychotic patients and many patients with chronic pain without surgery.

PRIMARY SENSORY RECEPTIVE AREAS

Three primary receptive areas of the cortex contain the terminations of specific sensory nuclei of the thalamus. Fibers conveying visual impulses from the lateral geniculate body extend to the cortex of the lips of the *calcarine fissure* (area 17). A lesion here in one of the hemispheres produces contralateral hemianopia. Fibers from the medial geniculate body carry auditory impulses to the *anterior transverse gyrus,* known as Heschl's gyrus (area 41). Unilateral lesions of this area have little effect because both ears have remaining connections to the intact temporal lobe. The ventral posterior nucleus relays tactile and proprioceptive impulses to the *postcentral gyrus,* which is the *primary somesthetic area* (areas 3, 2, and 1). Sensations of touch, pressure, and position are impaired on the opposite side of the body after unilateral lesions in this area, but pain and temperature sensations are not abolished. These sensations are perceived at the level of the thalamus. In the postcentral gyrus, as in the precentral gyrus, the face is represented ventrolaterally and the leg dorsomedially.

SECONDARY SENSORY AREAS

Near each primary receptive area are cortical zones that receive sensory inputs directly or indirectly from the thalamus. These secondary sensory areas contain somatotopic representations of parts of the body, but the areas are smaller than the primary areas and the order of representation is different. A secondary somatic sensory area is located along the superior lip of the lateral fissure. Parts of the body are represented there bilaterally, although the contralateral representation predominates. This area is involved in the perception of several sensory modalities, including touch, pressure, position sense, and pain. A secondary auditory area is located ventral to the primary auditory area, and a secondary visual area is contained within area 18.

Before sensory information can be comprehended fully, it must undergo elaboration and analysis in an extensive cortical zone adjacent to the primary sensory area, the *sensory association area.*

SENSORY ASSOCIATION AREAS

The *somesthetic* association area lies next to the postcentral gyrus in the parietal lobe (areas 5 and 7); the *visual* association area surrounds the visual area on the medial and lateral aspects of the occipital lobe (areas 18 and 19); and the *auditory* association area occupies a part of the superior temporal gyrus (areas 42 and 22) near the auditory area (see Figs. 50 and 51). The supramarginal (area 40) and angular (area 39) gyri also are important association areas that interrelate somesthetic, visual, and auditory stimuli. These association areas have the tasks of formulating sensory stimuli into object images and of comprehending their meaning. The process of comprehension ("knowing" or "gnosis") must entail a comparison of present sensory phenomena with past experience. For example, the visual association areas must be called upon when an old friend is recognized in a crowd. *Agnosia* is a failure to recognize stimuli when the appropriate sensory systems are functioning adequately. Agnosia commonly occurs in visual, tactile, and auditory forms.

Visual agnosia is the failure to recognize objects visually in the absence of a defect of visual acuity or intellectual impairment. The patient often can see the object clearly but cannot recognize or identify it visually. The same object usually can be identified by other sensibilities such as touch. Lesions of areas 18 and 19 in the dominant cerebral hemisphere usually are associated with visual agnosia.

Tactile agnosia is the inability to recognize objects by touch when tactile and proprioceptive sensibilities are intact in the part of the body being tested. Lesions of the supramarginal gyrus (area 40) of the dominant cerebral hemisphere usually are responsible for tactile agnosia. Patients with tactile agnosia often have disturbances of body image. They may not recognize individual fingers and may confuse the left and right sides of the body.

Auditory agnosia is the failure of a patient with intact hearing to recognize what he hears, including speech, musical sounds, or familiar noises. Bilateral lesions of the posterior part of the superior temporal convolution (area 22) are responsible.

The auditory and visual association zones border upon an extensive area of the temporal lobe in which visual and auditory sensory experiences apparently are placed in storage as if they had been permanently recorded on sound film. It is here that the unknown mechanisms of memory, hallucinations, and dreams may be located. By stimulating an isolated point of the superior temporal gyrus in conscious patients, neurosurgeons have been able to evoke detailed and vivid remembrances of specific, but unimportant, events that took place several years previously. Epileptic seizures caused by focal irritation in the temporal lobe may be ushered in by hallucinations of sound. Occasionally they are preceded by memory disturbances in which present and past experiences are confused so that an event of the present seems to be a repetition of something that has happened before, the *déjà vu* phenomenon. Memory recording is temporarily suspended during a temporal lobe seizure. The patient may continue to carry out purposive movements, but he remains amnesic for the attack. A further indication of the importance of the temporal lobes in memory function is that removal of both lobes in humans permanently abolishes the ability to store new information (i.e., to form new memories).

Apraxia, Aphasia, Alexia, and Agraphia

Apraxia is loss of the ability to carry out correctly certain movements in response to stimuli that normally excite them, in the absence of weakness, other motor disorders, or sensory loss, and with an intact comprehension of language. Accomplishing a complex act requires the integrity of a large part of the cerebral cortex. There must first be an idea—a mental formulation of the plan. This formulation must then be transferred by association fibers to the motor system where it can be executed. Apraxias often result from lesions interrupting connections between the site of formulation of a motor act and the motor areas responsible for its execution. A lesion of the supramarginal gyrus of the dominant parietal lobe leads to an *ideomotor apraxia,* in which a patient knows what he wants to do, but is unable to do it. He can perform many complex acts automatically, but cannot carry out the same acts on command. *Ideational apraxia* refers to failures in carrying out sequences of acts, although individual movements are correct. This form of apraxia results from lesions in the dominant parietal lobe or the corpus callosum. *Kinetic apraxia* (inability to execute fine acquired movements) and *gait apraxia* often result from disease of the frontal lobe. Apraxia may occur also with generalized cerebral cortical disease.

Facile use of language and speech is a remarkable attribute of the human brain—one that is shared by no other animal. Language refers to the vocabulary and syntactic rules needed for communication, regardless of the mode of production or comprehension. Speech refers to the production of spoken language. *Aphasia* is a disorder of language owing to a defect in either the production or comprehension of vocabulary or syntax. Beginning early in life, nearly every individual trains one hemisphere of the brain more intensively than the other in the processes of language function. It is usually the left side of the brain that assumes the leading role, and, in consequence, the person becomes right-handed. Right-handedness indicates the preferential use of the right hand in most or all unimanual activities. *Aphasia appears only if a lesion is located in the dominant hemisphere.* Dominance occurs relatively late in development. Thus a right-handed child of five who suffers an injury in the left hemisphere will learn to speak perfectly again in a year or two. An adult cannot recover to this extent.

Three regions of the dominant cerebral hemisphere are important in aphasia: Broca's area, Wernicke's area, and the intervening area of parietal lobe (the parietal operculum). Broca's area, the anterior speech region, is located on the motor cortex in the inferior frontal gyrus just rostral to the site of the motor representation of the face (Fig. 54). Wernicke's area lies in the posterior part of the superior temporal gyrus on the convexity of the brain and extends onto the upper surface of the temporal lobe. Wernicke's area is connected with Broca's area through the arcuate fasciculus, a fiber bundle coursing from the temporal lobe around the posterior end of the Sylvian fissure into the lower parietal lobe, running forward into the frontal lobe. The function of Wernicke's area is to make the individual capable of recognizing speech patterns relayed from the left primary auditory cortex. Information about incoming speech patterns is relayed to Broca's area, which generates the proper pattern of signals to the speech musculature for the production of sounds. Three general forms of aphasia are recognized that relate to Broca's area, Wernicke's area, and the parietal operculum.

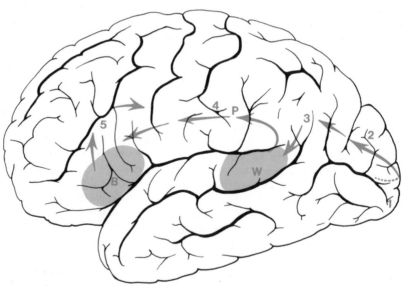

FIGURE 54. Cerebral cortical areas important in language. (W = Wernicke's region; B = Broca's region; P = parietal operculum.) A visual image is projected from the calcarine cortex (1) into the visual association areas 18 and 19 (2) to the region of the angular gyrus (3). Information is then transferred to Wernicke's area to arouse the learned auditory form of the object. This information is then transferred via the arcuate fasciculus (4) under the parietal operculum (P) to Broca's area (B), which contains programs that control (5) the cortical motor region involved in speech in the precentral gyrus.

Lesions of Broca's area lead to an executive (also termed motor, non-fluent, anterior, or Broca's) aphasia (see Fig. 54). The patient produces spoken language slowly and effortfully with poorly produced sounds and agrammatic, telegraphic speech. Many prepositions, nouns, and verbs are deleted. The patient has extreme difficulty in expressing certain grammatical words and phrases. "No ifs, ands, or buts" is a particularly difficult phrase to speak. The patient has good comprehension of spoken and written language but is frustrated and discouraged by his difficulty with speech. Vascular lesions of Broca's area often involve the internal capsule. Consequently, a right hemiplegia often accompanies an executive aphasia.

Lesions of Wernicke's area lead to a receptive (also termed sensory, fluent, posterior, or Wernicke's) aphasia (see Fig. 54). The patient produces spoken language more rapidly than normal, with normal grammatic construction. The patient cannot find the correct words to express his thoughts, however, and may omit words, use circumlocutions, use words without precise meanings, or substitute words. Substitutions of one word for another are called *verbal paraphasias*. *Literal paraphasias* are the substitution of a well-articulated but inappropriate phoneme in a word (e.g., saying pork for cork). Words may be produced that are random collections of sounds, and these are termed *neologisms*. The patient has poor comprehension of speech but generally can repeat spoken language. The patient often is unaware of his speech difficulty and may show no concern about it. Since lesions of Wernicke's area are far removed from the primary motor area and the internal capsule, patients with receptive aphasia usually are not also hemiplegic.

Lesions of the parietal operculum lead to a conduction aphasia by disconnecting Wernicke's area from Broca's area. The patient has a fluent aphasia with poor repetition of spoken language. Despite his phonetic errors, the patient tends to have good comprehension of spoken language.

Patients with posteriorly placed vascular lesions affecting speech may have damage to the angular gyrus associated with injury to Wernicke's area. Infarction of the angular gyrus of the dominant hemisphere results in loss of the ability to read (alexia) and write (agraphia).

The Internal Capsule

Afferent and efferent fibers of all parts of the cerebral cortex converge toward the brain stem, forming the *corona radiata* deep in the medullary substance of the hemisphere. As these fibers course ventrally from the cortex, the rostral ones pass down between the head of the caudate and the rostral end of the lentiform nucleus. These fibers form the *anterior limb of the internal capsule*. Caudally, the fibers pass between the thalamus and the lentiform nucleus as the *posterior limb* of the internal capsule. At the level of the interventricular foramen, the transition between the anterior and posterior limbs is called the genu (knee) of the internal capsule (see Fig. 55). Descending fibers of the pyramidal system pass through the posterior

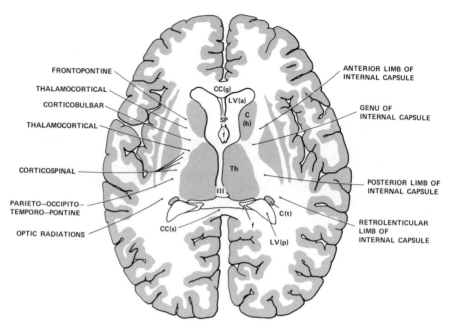

FIGURE 55. A horizontal section through the cerebrum to show the location of the internal capsule fibers (labeled on the right) and the various fiber bundles that make up the capsule (identified on the left). CC(g) = corpus callosum, genu; CC(s) = corpus callosum, splenium; C(h) = caudate head; C(t) = caudate tail; f = fornix; LV(a) = lateral ventricle, anterior horn; LV(p) = lateral ventricle, posterior horn; P = putamen; SP = septum pellucidum; Th = thalamus; III = third ventricle.

limb of the internal capsule. The corticobulbar fibers for movements of the muscles of the head are located rostral to the corticospinal fibers. Motor fibers to the upper extremity are rostral to those to the lower extremity. Fibers passing to and from the frontal lobe, other than pyramidal fibers, make up the anterior limb of the capsule, while those of the parietal lobe occupy the posterior part of the posterior limb. Optic radiation fibers are located in the retrolenticular portion of the internal capsule. Auditory radiation fibers are found in the sublenticular part of the internal capsule, which is below the plane of section of the brain slice pictured in Figure 55.

THE CEREBRAL ARTERIES

The *middle cerebral artery* (Fig. 56), a terminal branch of the internal carotid, enters the depth of the lateral fissure and divides into cortical branches that spread in a radiating fashion to supply the insula and the lateral surface of the frontal, parietal, occipital, and temporal lobes. The lateral and medial striate arteries, sometimes termed the lenticulostriate arteries, are small branches, variable in position and arrangement, which come from the basal part of the middle cerebral artery to supply the internal capsule and portions of the basal ganglia (Figs. 56 and 57). In the presence of arteriosclerosis and high blood pressure, one of the branches may rupture and cause hemorrhage into the substance of the internal capsule. The sudden collapse that such an accident produces is commonly spoken of as a "stroke," though this term also is used for the results of occlusion of a cerebral vessel without hemorrhage (ischemic infarction). A relatively small hemorrhage in the internal capsule may result in complete paralysis of the opposite side of the body because all corticospinal fibers are contained in one small area. Initially the patient has a hypotonic hemiplegia with decreased muscle stretch reflexes, and with time the patient develops a spastic hemiplegia with increased muscle stretch reflexes and an extensor plantar response. Sensory loss also may be produced if thalamocortical fibers to the parietal lobe are included. Large hemorrhages often are fatal, but after a less severe insult, the patient survives and may regain partial use of his limbs.

An occlusion of the main trunk of the middle cerebral artery by the formation of a clot *(thrombosis)* produces paralysis of the opposite side of the body with a preponderant effect in the face and upper extremity, hypesthesia in the same regions, and aphasia (if located in the dominant hemisphere). When individual cortical branches are occluded, the symptoms are

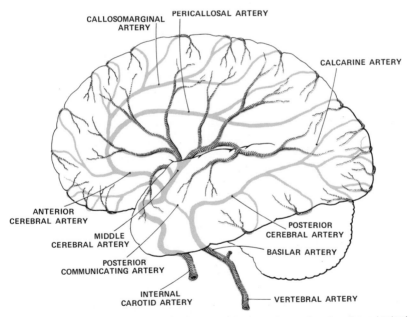

FIGURE 56. A left lateral view of the cerebral hemisphere, showing the principal arteries. The anterior cerebral and posterior cerebral arteries are on the medial surface and are shown as if projected through the substance of the brain.

limited to the loss of function in that particular region. For example, if the inferior frontal branch on the left is occluded, weakness will be noted in the lower part of the right face and tongue and the patient will have Broca's aphasia.

The *anterior cerebral artery,* a terminal branch of the internal carotid, turns medially to enter the median longitudinal cerebral fissure. On reaching the genu of the corpus callosum, it curves dorsally and turns backward close to the body of the corpus callosum, supplying branches to the medial surface of the frontal and parietal lobes, and also to an adjoining strip of cortex along the medial edge of the lateral surface of these lobes (see Figs. 56 and 57). A small recurrent branch (medial striate), given off near the base of the artery, supplies the anterior limb and genu of the internal capsule. Thrombosis along the course of the anterior cerebral artery produces paresis and hypesthesia of the opposite lower extremity.

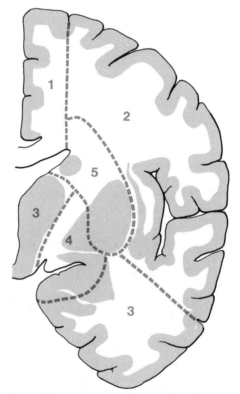

FIGURE 57. A cross section through the brain at about the level of the central sulcus, showing the areas of distribution of (1) the anterior cerebral artery; (2) the middle cerebral artery; (3) the posterior cerebral artery; (4) the medial striate arteries; and (5) the lateral striate arteries.

The basilar artery, a continuation of the fused vertebral arteries, bifurcates at the rostral border of the pons to form the *posterior cerebral arteries.* These arteries curve dorsally around the cerebral peduncles and send branches to the medial and inferior aspects of the temporal lobe, and to the occipital lobe (see Figs. 56 and 57). A separate branch, the calcarine artery, supplies the visual cortex. A number of perforating branches are given off that supply the posterior and lateral parts of the thalamus and the subthalamus (see Fig. 57). Occlusion of the thalamic branches produces hemiplegia with complete loss of sensation in the opposite limbs. In time the *thalamic syndrome* appears, consisting of severe, constant pain in the hemiplegic limbs. The pain is agonizing and often has a burning quality. Sensations of touch, pain, and temperature are decreased in the affected limbs. In addition to the sensory changes, symptoms of cerebellar asynergia and tremor may be produced in the extremities of the opposite side from damage to fibers of the superior cerebellar peduncle ascending to the ventral lateral nucleus of the thalamus. The calcarine branch of the posterior cerebral artery may be occluded independently of the thalamic branches. In this case the only sign produced will be contralateral hemianopia. Bilateral occlusion of the posterior cerebral arteries can lead to a deficit of memory because of injury to the temporal lobes bilaterally.

Circulus Arteriosus and Central Branches

The *circulus arteriosus* (circle of Willis) is formed by the junction of the basilar artery and the two internal carotid arteries through the presence of a pair of posterior communicating arteries and an anterior communicating artery. (The communicating arteries vary considerably between people, and Figure 58 purposely shows one posterior vessel somewhat smaller.) All the major cerebral vessels have their origin from the arterial circle.

The central arteries supply the structures within the interior of the brain: the diencephalon, corpus striatum, and internal capsule. These vessels are branches of the arterial circle and may be conveniently considered in four groups:

1. The *anterior medial group* originates from the anterior cerebral and anterior communicating arteries. Distribution involves the anterior perforated substance to supply the anterior hypothalamic region (preoptic and supraoptic regions).
2. The *posterior medial group* originates from the posterior cerebral and posterior communicating arteries. Distribution involves the posterior perforated substance. The rostral group supplies the tuber cinereum, stalk, and hypophysis. Deeper branches penetrate the thalamus. The caudal group supplies the mammillary bodies, subthalamus, and medial portions of the thalamus and midbrain.
3. The *anterior lateral group* originates primarily from the middle cerebral arteries; the *medial striate* or *anterior recurrent* vessels origi-

nate from the anterior cerebral arteries. Distribution involves the anterior perforated substance. The medial striate vessels supply the anterior limb and genu of the internal capsule. The lateral striate vessels supply the basal ganglia and the anterior limb of the internal capsule. These vessels are also known as lenticulostriate arteries.

4. The *posterior lateral group* originates from the posterior cerebral artery. Distribution involves the caudal portion of the thalamus (geniculate bodies, pulvinar and lateral nuclei).

The anterior and posterior choroidal arteries are considered to be central branches. The anterior vessel arises from the middle cerebral artery and supplies the choroid plexus of the lateral ventricles, the hippocampus, some of the globus pallidus, and the posterior limb of the internal capsule (see Fig. 57). The posterior choroidal artery arises from the posterior cerebral artery and supplies the choroid plexus of the third ventricle and the dorsal surface of the thalamus.

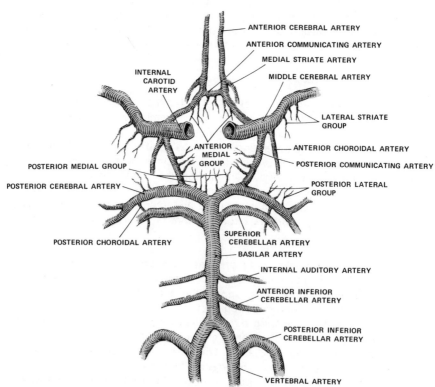

FIGURE 58. A diagram illustrating the origin of the branches from the circulus arteriosus (circle of Willis).

Angiography

Angiography or arteriography refers to the general procedure in which arteries of the brain are studied by x-ray following injection of the vessels with radiopaque material. The internal carotid or the vertebral arteries serve as the usual site of injection. Commonly a catheter will be placed in a femoral or brachial artery and threaded into one of these arteries in the neck.

Cerebral angiography has been useful in determining the site of aneurysms and any anomalous development of the larger branches of the cerebral arterial circle. Cerebral hemorrhage, infarction, tumors, and vascular spasm often may be localized by the finding of an alteration in the arterial pattern. Generally, the smaller terminal arteries are not identified by cerebral arteriography. Injection of the internal carotid artery outlines the anterior and middle cerebral arteries. The major branches of the basilar artery (cerebellar and posterior cerebral arteries) are outlined following injection of the vertebral artery. The posterior communicating artery, if it is sizable, may be apparent following either injection.

24

THE BASAL GANGLIA
AND RELATED STRUCTURES

Motor activity is intricately controlled by the interaction of three major systems: the cerebral cortex, the cerebellum, and the basal ganglia. The cerebral cortex exerts its influence on the lower motoneurons either directly through the *pyramidal system* (corticospinal and corticobulbar tracts), or indirectly through polysynaptic, *extrapyramidal pathways,* such as the corticoreticulospinal tract and the corticorubrospinal tract (see Chapter 4). In addition, the basal ganglia and the cerebellum influence motor function, but in the human brain their major influence is exerted by their projections to the motor cortex. Thus the pyramidal and extrapyramidal systems are so closely interconnected that a distinction is meaningless. Nevertheless, the term extrapyramidal system is frequently used clinically to denote the components of the basal ganglia and related subcortical nuclei that influence motor activity.

STRUCTURES IN THE BASAL GANGLIA

The interrelations of the structures in the basal ganglia are complex, and the terminology used in describing these structures can be confusing. A thorough understanding of the terminology is an essential prerequisite for understanding the interconnections of this system.

The major components of the basal ganglia include the *caudate nucleus,* the *putamen,* and the *globus pallidus.* Although some authorities include the amygdaloid nuclear complex and the claustrum, they will not be considered in this discussion. Two other subcortical nuclei, the *subthalamic nucleus and the substantia nigra,* are not specifically part of the basal ganglia per se, but are functionally related. Table 2 provides a guide to the terminology associated with this system. Reference to the table should make it apparent that "nigrostriatal" is a proper name for a pathway that arises in the substantia nigra and terminates in the putamen, the caudate nucleus, or in both. Similarly, "pallidosubthalamic" is an appropriate name for a pathway that arises in the globus pallidus and projects to the subthalamic nucleus. Note that "corpus striatum" and "striatum" are not synonymous terms. They are frequently mistaken to be equivalent.

The *caudate nucleus* occupies a position in the floor of the lateral ventricle, dorsolateral to the thalamus (Fig. 59). The bulge at the cephalic end of the caudate is known as the *head.* The *body* passes backward at the side of the thalamus and tapers gradually to form the *tail,* which curves ventrally and follows the inferior horn of the lateral ventricle into the temporal lobe, ending near the amygdala. Some authorities divide the caudate nucleus merely into a head and a tail.

The *lenticular,* or *lentiform, nucleus* (see Fig. 59) is a thumb-sized mass wedged against the lateral side of the internal capsule. It is separated from the caudate nucleus by fibers of the internal capsule except in the cephalic part where these two nuclear masses fuse around the border of the anterior limb of the capsule. The lenticular nucleus is divided into the *putamen* and the *globus pallidus.* The putamen is the lateral portion and has the same histologic appearance as the caudate nucleus. The globus pallidus, in the

TABLE 2. Basal Ganglia Nomenclature

| TERM | DESCRIPTIVE TERMS | | SYNONYM | COMPONENTS |
	PREFIX	SUFFIX		
Striatum	Strio-	-striate -striate	Neostriatum	Caudate and Putamen
Pallidum	Pallido-	-pallidal	Paleostriatum	Globus Pallidus
Lenticular Nucleus				Putamen and Globus Pallidus
Corpus Striatum				Caudate, Putamen, and Globus Pallidus
Subthalamic Nucleus	Subthalamo-	-subthalamic		
Substantia Nigra	Nigro-	-nigral		Pars compacta and Pars reticularis

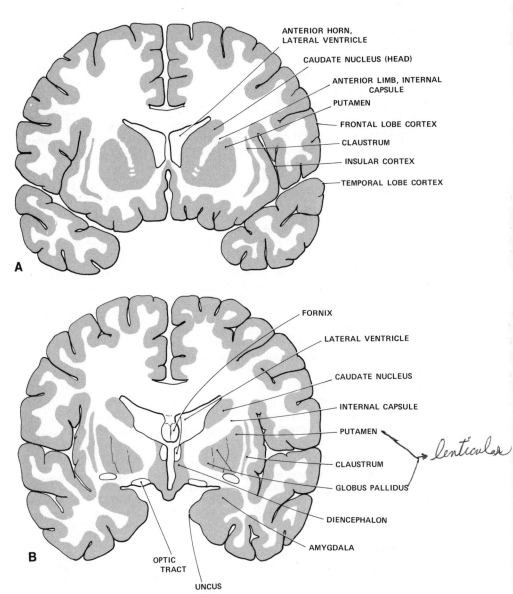

ANTERIOR HORN,
LATERAL VENTRICLE

CAUDATE NUCLEUS (HEAD)

ANTERIOR LIMB, INTERNAL
CAPSULE

PUTAMEN

FRONTAL LOBE CORTEX

CLAUSTRUM

INSULAR CORTEX

TEMPORAL LOBE CORTEX

A

FORNIX

LATERAL VENTRICLE

CAUDATE NUCLEUS

INTERNAL CAPSULE

PUTAMEN

CLAUSTRUM

GLOBUS PALLIDUS

DIENCEPHALON

AMYGDALA

OPTIC
TRACT

UNCUS

B

lenticular

FIGURE 59. Two coronal sections through the cerebral hemispheres. *A.* Section through the rostral part of the frontal lobe to show the relationship of the basal ganglia to the surrounding telencephalic structures. *B.* Section through the caudal part of the frontal lobe, showing the location of the basal ganglia lateral to the diencephalon.

medial region of the lenticular nucleus, contains more large cells and is traversed by many myelinated fibers, which accounts for its pale appearance in the fresh state.

The *subthalamus* is closely related to the basal ganglia in function and contains the *zona incerta* (located between the lenticular fasciculus and the thalamic fasciculus), *Forel's tegmental field H* (which includes the *prerubral field*), and the *subthalamic nucleus* (of Luys). The zona incerta and the scattered cells in the prerubral field are considered by some to be a rostral continuation of the midbrain reticular formation. The rostral portions of the *substantia nigra* and the *red nucleus* extend into the region. The *subthalamic nucleus,* lens-shaped and lying along the medial border of the internal capsule, is contiguous with the substantia nigra at its caudal extent.

CONNECTIONS OF THE BASAL GANGLIA

The major input to the basal ganglia is from the cerebral cortex. From neurons in all areas of the neocortex, axons project to the striatum (Figs. 60 and 61). The primary motor (area 4) and sensory (areas 3, 1, and 2) cortices show a preferential projection to the putamen, while association areas of the frontal, parietal, occipital, and temporal lobes project heavily onto the caudate nucleus. From the striatum fibers pass directly to the lateral and medial segments of the globus pallidus.

The major outflow of efferent fibers from the basal ganglia comes from the medial segment of the globus pallidus (see Fig. 61). Some of these fibers stream directly across the posterior limb of the internal capsule. Upon entering the subthalamic region they form a bundle known as the *lenticular fasciculus* (Forel's field H$_2$), located immediately ventral to the zona incerta (ZI). Another bundle of fibers from the globus pallidus (medial segment) passes around the ventral aspect of the posterior limb of the internal capsule to form a loop, the *ansa lenticularis*. Both bundles merge on the medial aspect of the ZI in the prerubral field where cerebellothalamic fibers join them. The bundles then curve dorsally and pass laterally just dorsal to the ZI to form a discrete bundle called the *thalamic fasciculus* (Forel's field H$_1$). The fibers in these systems synapse in the *centromedian, ventral lateral,* and *ventral anterior* nuclei of the thalamus. A third bundle of efferent fibers (the *pallidosubthalamic fibers*) arises from the globus pallidus (but in this case, primarily from the lateral segment), crosses the posterior limb of the internal capsule, and synapses in the subthalamic nucleus. The cells of this nucleus, in turn, project back to the globus pallidus, but primarily to the medial segment. Finally, a fourth bundle arises from the medial segment of the globus pallidus and descends as *pallidotegmental fibers* to terminate in the *pedunculopontine tegmental nucleus* in the caudal aspect of the midbrain. The latter bundle is the only pathway that arises from the basal ganglia to descend caudal to the level of the substantia nigra.

The *substantia nigra* is a subcortical nucleus that is very closely related to the basal ganglia (see Fig. 60). It is reciprocally connected with the

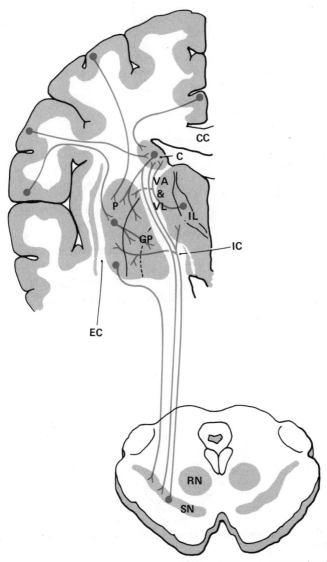

FIGURE 60. The afferent and efferent connections of the caudate and putamen. C = caudate nucleus; CC = corpus callosum; EC = external capsule; GP = globus pallidus; IC = internal capsule; IL = intralaminar nuclei of the thalamus; P = putamen; RN = red nucleus; SN = substantia nigra; VA = ventral anterior nucleus of the thalamus; VL = ventral lateral nucleus of the thalamus.

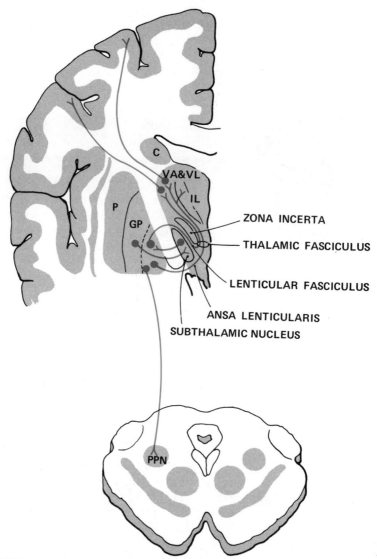

FIGURE 61. The efferent connections of the globus pallidus. PPN = pedunculo-pontine tegmental nucleus.

striatum and sends efferents to the *ventral anterior* and, to some extent, to the *ventral lateral* thalamic nuclei. Neurons that arise in the pars compacta of the substantia nigra transmit dopamine, an inhibitory substance, to the striatum, while the nigrothalamic projections arise from nondopaminergic cells in the pars reticulata.

There are many circuits and feedback loops within and between the structures related to the basal ganglia. One very significant circuit is the following: cerebral cortex → striatum → globus pallidus → thalamus → cerebral cortex. Another loop includes: cortex → striatum → substantia nigra → thalamus → cortex. Many smaller circuits exist between structures that have reciprocal connections (for example, substantia nigra ⇌ striatum, and subthalamic nucleus ⇌ pallidum).

The basal ganglia and the cerebellum interact with the cerebral cortex through a series of feedback circuits. The dentate and interposed nuclei of the cerebellum project to the ventrolateral nucleus of the thalamus, which also receives projections from the globus pallidus and the substantia nigra. Recent evidence indicates that none of these projections overlaps in the ventrolateral nucleus. The ventrolateral nucleus projects to the primary motor region of the cerebral cortex. In turn, the motor cortex (and other regions of the cerebrum) projects to the striatum to enter the basal ganglia circuit; moreover, it projects to the pons to enter the cerebellar circuit, including the corticopontocerebellar tract, Purkinje cells, interposed and dentate nuclei, and the cerebellothalamic tract. Consequently, both systems influence the part of the cerebral cortex that gives rise to the descending motor pathways (pyramidal and "extrapyramidal"), which affect the activity of the lower motoneurons.

FUNCTIONAL CONSIDERATIONS

Parkinson's disease, or paralysis agitans, is a common condition associated with degenerative changes (neuronal degeneration and depigmentation) in the substantia nigra and locus ceruleus. The pathologic changes in the substantia nigra lead to the depletion of dopamine in the caudate nucleus and putamen, owing to loss of nigrostriatal neuronal connections. Patients with Parkinson's disease develop akinesia, rigidity, and tremor. The akinesia is manifested as difficulty in initiating and performing volitional movements of the most common type, including standing, walking, eating, and writing. The lines of the patient's face are smooth, his expression is fixed (the so-called masked face), and there is no spontaneous emotional response. The patient stands with head and shoulders stooped and walks with short, shuffling steps. The arms are held at the sides and do not swing in rhythm with the legs, as they should, automatically. Although the patient has difficulty in starting to take the first steps, once under way the pace becomes more and more rapid, and the patient has trouble in stopping his progress when he reaches his goal. Rigidity of the limbs (i.e., increased resistance to passive movement) is present in most patients with Parkinson's disease and often consists of "cogwheel" rigidity. When the examiner passively flexes or extends one of the patient's extremities, an increased resistance occurs that suddenly gives way and then returns sequentially as the movement continues, in the manner of a cogwheel. The muscle stretch (deep tendon) reflexes usually are normal. The tremor of Parkinson's disease usually occurs with the patient at rest and consists of

4- to 6-cycle-per-second flexion-extension movements of the fingers and wrists, at times in the form of a "pill-rolling" movement. Treatment of Parkinson's disease consists of the administration of drugs that enhance the dopaminergic activity of the basal ganglia. Surgical therapy, consisting of the placement of a lesion in the globus pallidus or ventrolateral nucleus of the thalamus, has been used extensively in the past and now is reserved generally for patients who fail to respond to medical therapy.

Chorea is a movement disorder resulting from disease of the basal ganglia. Choreiform movements consist of a rapid, irregular flow of motions, including "piano-playing" flexion-extension movements of the fingers, elevation and depression of the shoulders and hips, crossing and uncrossing of the legs, and grimacing movements of the face. Hemichorea consists of choreiform movements limited to one side of the body, usually resulting from a vascular lesion of the contralateral basal ganglia. The disorder usually occurs abruptly in middle age and often is accompanied by weakness of the affected limbs. Sydenham's chorea occurs in children as a complication of rheumatic fever, but the disease is self-limited and recovery is complete. Huntington's disease is an inherited disorder characterized by progressive dementia and choreiform movements, usually beginning in adult life. There are marked degenerative changes in the cerebral cortex and basal ganglia, particularly in the caudate nucleus and putamen.

Athetosis is a movement disorder characterized by slow, writhing movements of a wormlike character involving the extremities, trunk, and neck. Athetosis often occurs in association with dystonia, which is the abnormal persistence of limb and trunk postures. Athetosis is seen frequently in patients with cerebral palsy and results from brain damage that occurred at or prior to birth.

Hemiballismus is a movement disorder characterized by the sudden onset of continuous, wild, flinging motions of the arm and leg on one side of the body. This results most often from a vascular lesion of the contralateral subthalamic nucleus.

25

THE CEREBROSPINAL FLUID

The brain and spinal cord are suspended in cerebrospinal fluid, a clear, watery liquid that fills the subarachnoid space surrounding them. The four ventricles of the brain also are filled with this fluid. The average total quantity of fluid in adults is estimated to be 130 cc. It is constantly being renewed by production and reabsorption so that the total volume is replaced several times daily. Small amounts of protein, sugar, electrolytes, and a very few lymphocytes (no more than 3 per cu mm) are present in the fluid. Its general composition is that of an ultrafiltrate of blood with some constituents added through secretion.

FORMATION AND CIRCULATION OF CEREBROSPINAL FLUID

The cerebrospinal fluid is formed mainly by the *choroid plexuses*, which are tufts of dilated capillaries that project into the walls of the ventricles in certain regions. There are two large plexuses, one in the floor of each lateral ventricle, supplemented by smaller ones in the roofs of the third and fourth ventricles.

There is slow movement of fluid from the ventricles into the subarachnoid spaces from which it is shunted into the dural venous sinuses and removed by the blood stream. The fluid leaves the lateral ventricles through the *interventricular foramina* (foramina of Munro), traverses the third ventricle, and reaches the fourth ventricle by way of the *cerebral aqueduct*—the narrowest passageway of its entire route (Fig. 62). Three openings in the fourth ventricle allow the cerebrospinal fluid to pass from the ventricles into the subarachnoid space outside the brain. The two *lateral ventricular foramina* (foramina of Luschka) are located in the lateral recesses of the fourth ventricle; the *median ventricular foramen* (foramen of Magendie) is in the midline of the roof of the fourth ventricle. The subarachnoid space, which lies between the arachnoid membrane externally and the pia mater internally, provides a route by which the fluid can flow from its site of production in the ventricles to the points of absorption. Cerebrospinal fluid flows from the outlet foramina of the fourth ventricle over the whole surface of the brain and spinal cord. In places where the brain surface is not close to the bone of the skull, small pockets of cerebrospinal fluid are found within the subarachnoid space, particularly around the base of the brain. The largest of these is the *cisterna magna* between the inferior surface of the cerebellum and the medulla. Other cisterns—the pontine, interpeduncular, and chiasmatic—lie between the base of the brain and the floor of the cranial cavity. The *cisterna superior* (cisterna ambiens) is the pocket of fluid that lies dorsal to the midbrain.

Spinal fluid fills the tubular extension of the subarachnoid space, which forms a sleeve around the spinal cord. The lower limit of this space is variable, but on the average it lies at the body of the second sacral vertebra, considerably below the end of the spinal cord. Although the spinal subarachnoid space is, in effect, a blind pocket, exchange of spinal fluid takes place by a slow mixing process induced by changes in posture.

Cerebrospinal fluid diffuses upward from the basal areas of the brain over the convexities of the hemispheres until it reaches the *arachnoid villi* in the walls of the superior sagittal sinus. It is absorbed through these villi into the venous blood stream in the sinus. A small amount may be absorbed from the subarachnoid space surrounding the spinal cord by the vessels in the sheaths of emerging nerves. The veins and capillaries of the pia mater also may be capable of removing some cerebrospinal fluid.

The subarachnoid space extends into the substance of the nervous system through extensions around blood vessels known as perivascular, or *Virchow-Robin,* spaces. Every blood vessel entering the nervous system passes across the subarachnoid space and carries with it a sleeve of arachnoid immediately surrounding the vessel and a sleeve of pia mater more externally. The cerebrospinal fluid of the subarachnoid space probably receives a contribution from the perivascular spaces. Within the depths of the central nervous system the layers of pia and arachnoid fuse so that the perivascular space does not continue to the level of the capillary beds.

PRESSURE OF CEREBROSPINAL FLUID

Any obstruction to the normal passage of cerebrospinal fluid causes the fluid to back up in the ventricles and leads to a general increase of intracra-

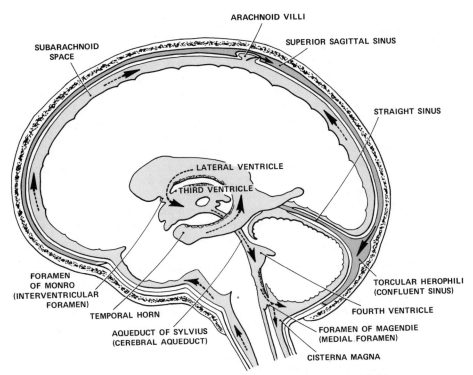

FIGURE 62. A diagram illustrating the circulation of the cerebrospinal fluid.

nial pressure. After the pressure has been elevated for some time, usually a matter of days or weeks, the effect can be seen by inspecting the fundus of the eye with an ophthalmoscope. Due to the high pressure inside the sleeve of dura mater that surrounds the optic nerve, the retinal veins are dilated and the optic nerve head (optic disk) is pushed forward above the level of the retina. This is known as *papilledema,* or *choked disk.* If papilledema has persisted for a long time, the fibers of the optic nerve will be damaged and the disk assumes a chalk-white color instead of the normal pale pink.

The most common cause of papilledema is a tumor of the brain compressing some part of the ventricular system. Tumors far removed from the ventricles may not produce obstruction until they reach very large size. A tumor of the cerebellum generally exerts pressure on the roof of the fourth ventricle, and, since it is confined within the posterior fossa by the semirigid tentorium cerebelli with little room for expansion, it is likely to cause early obstruction to the flow of cerebrospinal fluid through the fourth ventricle. Tumors near the orbital surface of one frontal lobe may compress the optic nerve and produce optic atrophy in the affected eye, while the other eye develops papilledema from generalized elevation of pressure as the tumor expands in size, a condition known as the Foster Kennedy syndrome. Other cardinal signs of brain tumor, in addition to papilledema, are persistent headache and vomiting. The headache probably results from the stretching of nerve endings in the dura mater and intracranial blood vessels. The cause of the nausea and vomiting is not clear, but stimulation of the vagal nuclei in the floor of the fourth ventricle may be involved.

Hydrocephalus is an increase in the volume of cerebrospinal fluid within the skull. It can occur with or without an increase in pressure. Hydrocephalus without an increase in pressure is termed *compensatory hydrocephalus* or *hydrocephalus ex vacuo*. In most cases it represents an increase in the volume of cerebrospinal fluid as a compensation for cerebral atrophy due to a primary central nervous system disease. Hydrocephalus with increased pressure can be subdivided into *obstructive hydrocephalus* and *communicating hydrocephalus*. Obstructive hydrocephalus results from an obstacle to the circulation of cerebrospinal fluid within the ventricles, the aqueduct, or at the outlet of the fourth ventricle. The result is loss of communication between the ventricles and the subarachnoid space, with a consequent increase in fluid within the ventricular system. Many types of pathology may cause obstructive hydrocephalus, including brain tumors, inflammatory processes, and developmental abnormalities. In communicating hydrocephalus there is free communication between the ventricles and the subarachnoid space. Hydrocephalus results either from a disturbance in the production and absorption of cerebrospinal fluid or from an obstruction to its circulation in the subarachnoid space.

Samples of cerebrospinal fluid for diagnostic tests are obtained by directing a long needle between two lumbar vertebrae below the level of L_2 and inserting it far enough to reach and pierce the dura mater. There is only slight danger of injuring the nerve roots of the cauda equina that are present at this level. With the patient relaxed and in a recumbent position, the pressure of the spinal fluid should not exceed 200 mm of water. Small oscillations of the fluid level in a manometer connected to the needle arise from the transmission of the cerebral pulse. These pulsations indicate that free communication is present. If blockage of the spinal subarachnoid space is suspected, the *Queckenstedt test* can be performed. With the needle in place and a water manometer attached, the jugular veins are compressed for 10 seconds. Under normal conditions there will be a rapid rise and fall in pressure, normal levels returning within a few seconds. In patients with obstruction of the subarachnoid space in the region of the foramen magnum or within the spinal canal, the rise of pressure from jugular compression is slight or absent. The Queckenstedt test should never be performed if symptoms of elevated intracranial pressure are present because of the danger of herniation of the cerebellar tonsils and the medulla through the foramen magnum. Even a lumbar puncture is hazardous in the presence of elevated intracranial pressure, since the release of pressure from below may allow similar herniation. Herniation of the medulla through the foramen magnum can cause death from injury to neurons controlling cardiac and respiratory function.

Spinal fluid also can be obtained by passing a needle at the base of the skull directly through the atlanto-occipital membrane into the cisterna magna. No nervous structures are encountered, but the needle will strike the medulla if it should slip too far. For this reason, cisternal puncture should be performed only under the supervision of experienced persons.

PNEUMOENCEPHALOGRAPHY AND COMPUTERIZED AXIAL TOMOGRAPHY

If the pineal body is calcified, its shadow may be seen in x-rays, and displacement in its position may yield significant information. Thinning or erosion of skull bones, as shown by x-ray, may help to establish the presence of a mass in the adjacent parts of the brain. Most tumors, however, cannot be visualized directly unless they are partly calcified. If the cerebrospinal fluid is completely withdrawn from the ventricular spaces and replaced by air, these spaces will appear as shadows in an x-ray. Dilations, distortions in shape, and filling defects can then be studied in considerable detail. This process, known as *pneumoencephalography*, is accomplished by means of lumbar puncture. If the intracranial pressure is increased, lumbar puncture cannot be performed safely, and it is necessary to introduce air directly into the ventricular system to obtain a visible outline by x-ray *ventriculography*. This process requires the drilling of trephine holes in the parietal bones through which needles can be passed into both lateral ventricles.

Computerized axial tomography (CAT) scanning is a recent advance that makes it possible to visualize many central nervous system structures without difficult and painful procedures such as pneumoencephalography and ventriculography. CAT scanning consists of passing x-rays through a patient's head from many different sites circumferentially and determining the degree of attenuation of the x-ray beams with a computer. The result is an image of the brain in cross section with a remarkable degree of detail. The CAT scan provides an image of the anatomy of the brain but gives no indication of its metabolic activity. A procedure now under development, positron emission tomography (PET) scanning, provides a noninvasive means of studying cerebral blood flow and metabolism.

INDEX

A *t* following a page number indicates a table.

XII tongue → ipsi lesion   ipsi

uvula → Nl side   contra

V chin → lesion   ipsi